Causal Inference

Epidemiology Resources Inc.

CAUSAL INFERENCE

edited by
Kenneth J. Rothman

Stephan F. Lanes
George N. Schlesinger
Mervyn Susser
Douglas L. Weed

Sander Greenland
Michael Jacobsen
Darwin R. Labarthe
Malcolm Maclure
Neil McIntyre
Diana B. Petitti
Charles Poole
Reuel A. Stallones

Epidemiology Resources Inc.
P.O. Box 339
Chestnut Hill, Massachusetts 02167.

Library of Congress Catalog Card number 87-22227
ISBN 0-917227-03-4

Printed in the United States of America

Cover design: Steiner + Schenkel Communication Design

Contents

COMMENT

REJOINDER

EDITOR'S INTRODUCTION

Inferring Causal Connections—
Habit, Faith or Logic?

Kenneth J. Rothman

Department of Family and Community Medicine
University of Massachusetts Medical School

The ability to infer causation is an essential survival trait. It is an ability that may be refined among reflective humans, but it is also one that can be identified in some form among other animals as well. Consider the example of my dog, a German shepherd who has learned to ring my doorbell when she wants to come into the house. This behavior was not actively taught, nor can I credit the idea that the dog observed others ringing the bell to go in and copied the behavior, especially since no visitor can approach the house when the dog is outside. Apparently this dog, which no one describes as being unusually bright, learned by herself that if she stands on her hind legs and presses the doorbell button with her paw, someone inside will open the door for her. Is this behavior simply an ironic twist to the classical Pavlovian experiment, with the dog ringing the bell and the people responding? Can we properly say that the dog has inferred, in some sense, that ringing the doorbell will cause her to be admitted, or should we describe the phenomenon merely as a conditioned behavior pattern, arising because the dog was reinforced for an exuberant lunge at the door? Indeed, what is the difference, if any?

Suppose one awakes with itchy red lesions distributed ubiquitously over one's skin. Yesterday one began a ten-day course of antibiotic therapy to control a sinus infection. It seems possible that the antibiotic has caused an allergic response. The antibiotic is known to cause allergic reactions, including skin rashes, in some people. Is a causal inference reasonable here? The rash might be caused by something in last night's dinner, poison ivy in the sheets, or any number of other possibilities. Even if no other possibility could be conjured up that seemed plausible, inferring a connection between the antibiotic and the rash might be wrong, because the cause of the rash could involve factors not perceived or imagined. Suppose, despite uncertainty, that the antibiotic were discontinued for awhile, and started again later. Suppose that this pattern were repeated many times, each time followed by the appearance of the rash. How many repetitions are needed to "establish" the causal connection? Do the repetitions constitute an empirical demonstration that serves as a valid platform for inference, or is the process still steeped in uncertainty? Is the inference different from the motivation of my dog in ringing the doorbell? Does the statement, surreptitiously inserted earlier in this paragraph, that "the antibiotic is known to cause allergic reactions" involve a different sort of inference from the one directed at explaining the occurrence of this one specific rash? What is meant by "known to cause allergic reactions" anyway? Is this certain knowledge or is it conjectural?

Such questions are not easy to answer. While philosophers have grappled with the task of understanding causal inference for a long time, and unquestionably made progress, many scientists who face the problem of making causal inferences have devoted little or no attention to developing a formal understanding of the process. Outside of the physical sciences, much of scientific knowledge comprises a collection of causal statements. The principles by which knowledge accumulates are the principles that describe the formulation and evaluation of those statements, and they constitute the subject of this book.

Since ancient times it has been recognized that some knowledge, such as mathematics, is self-contained, being based on an initial set of postulates and derived entirely from them without reference to empirical phenomena, whereas other knowledge draws on observations made of the real world. Classically, knowledge that was self-contained accumulated through a set of principles that we call deductive logic, which is a set of rules for deriving true conclusions from true premises. Of course, it is not surprising to hear of mathematical proofs that are retracted because critics discovered errors in the proof. When I asked Stephen Scheinberg, a mathematician friend of mine, how the validity of a proof is determined in mathematics, he responded pragmatically that when 90 per cent of mathematicians who examine the proof agree that it is correct, then it is considered a valid proof. This pragmatism is predicated on the rational abilities of mathematicians reviewing the proof. The averred uncertainty in establishing deductive proofs does not derive from the method itself, but only from error in the application of the rules.

Empirical knowledge, on the other hand, seems to accumulate through a different method, one that does not guarantee correct conclusions no matter how carefully it is employed. The fallibility of scientific knowledge about nature appears to be inherent in its dependence on observations, which are themselves fallible, and the inescapable limitation that observations are finite, and thus cannot take into account the infinity of conceivable circumstances in which the laws of nature might be applied. Induction, to use the term favored by early empiricists to describe the method by which repeated observations could "induce" the formulation of a law of nature, was shown to be an incomplete form of reasoning by David Hume, the British philosopher. The validity of induction has been an arena of contention ever since Hume, and it is a pivotal issue for the contributors of this volume. Hume pointed out that observers cannot perceive causal connections, but only a series of events. Even with multiple repetitions, the assignment of a causal interpretation or the formulation of a law of nature from the series of perceptions cannot be construed as a logical extension of the observations, despite our innate tendency to do so. Much of the philosophy of science since the time of Hume has been aimed either at justifying the use of induction in light of Hume's criticism, or attempting to understand the epistemology of science without induction. (Bertrand Russell noted wryly that "for a long time philosophers took care to be unintelligible, since otherwise everybody would have perceived that they had been unsuccessful in answering Hume."[1])

An understanding of the process of causal inference is often muddled by differing concepts of the term "inference" in empirical science, a problem that may reflect the uncertainty of the process itself. What passes for causal inference by scientists is often just decision-making perched upon weak criteria that lack a logical base. Many of the commonly used modes of causal inference are fallacious, their popularity notwithstanding. For example, one such method of inference, the method of "consensus," has been embraced, presumably for political reasons, by the National Institutes of Health. According to this method, a causal inference can be drawn when a consensus of experts knowledgeable about the issue is formed. The National Institutes of Health regularly convenes Consensus Development Conferences to address specific questions and draw inferences. The difficulty with this method is that consensus is no guarantee of correctness, as has been historically demonstrated in many instances. For one thing, consensus is temporary, and can change. Were consensus a correct basis for inference, then a once flat earth must have become spherical, and the thymus gland must have been physiologically inert until a couple of decades ago when it suddenly developed a useful role in the immune system. For another thing, consensus itself requires no further justification, and may be based on shared beliefs that are irrational. When *One Hundred Authors Against Einstein*, a collection of essays by 100 physicists attempting to discredit relativity theory, was published in 1930, Einstein reputedly responded to a reporter's query about the book with the remark: "Were my theory wrong, it would have taken but one person to show it." Similarly, it would require but one mathematician to point out a flaw in a deductive proof, despite consensus of other mathematicians that the proof is correct.

Another faulty approach to inference is to infer by "appeal to authority." While it would hardly seem to need saying that the seal of approval from a noted authority does not provide any logical basis for inference, in everyday practice many inferences are premised on little but the credentials of the theory's leading exponent. The flip side of an appeal to authority is the *ad hominem* criticism, which disallows an inferential argument simply because of the imagined lack of necessary credentials, or presumed biases, of the person who presents it. Of course, on reflection it seems obvious that an inference should stand or fall by virtue of its logic and the relevant data, and not by virtue of the imputed viewpoint, philosophy, personal biases, heritage or other interests of the person who puts forth the argument. As straightforward as this principle may seem, a trend in the biomedical literature is to encourage *ad hominem* evaluation by judging a work according to the affiliation or funding source of the researchers, rather than judging it by their findings or arguments. For example, in a review of a new method to interpret published results of clinical trials, Sacks et al.[2] criticized a majority of the analyses because they did not cite their source of support. Their comment was "We think that it is useful for the reader to know who supported a study, when deciding how much credence to give to its conclusions."[2] This statement baldly extols the use of prejudice to judge research, rather than judging the work on its merit. Interestingly, mandatory citation of funding source became a part of the publication policy of the New England Journal of Medicine in 1984, when the editor, concerned about possible conflicts of interest, noted that such citation "alerts readers to information they may wish to have as they assess the published report."[3] Some journals employ blind review of submitted papers by referees (that is, the identity of the authors is masked from the referees during the review) just to avoid *ad hominem* judgments, but judging a theory or a study according to the characteristics or presumed motives of the person or people who present it is still common practice.

Another fallacy in causal inference is the fallacy of *post hoc ergo propter hoc*, which is Latin for "after this therefore on-account-of this." It is a fallacy to infer that the rooster causes the sun to rise each morning by crowing at dawn, despite multiple repetitions of the same sequence of events. Although this fallacy is well recognized, the extension of a series of events observed repeatedly into a law of nature appears to be the backbone of the inductive method. Induction is still touted because it often seems to work. The difficulty is that in principle there is nothing behind the so-called logic of it but for the *post hoc* fallacy. Russell summarized the fallacy in this way:

> We have . . . the ordinary procedure of induction: 'If *p*, then *q*; now *q* is true; therefore *p* is true.' E.g., 'If pigs have wings, then some winged animals are good to eat; now some winged animals are good to eat; therefore pigs have wings.' This form of inference is called 'scientific method.'[4]

How can we differentiate between instances in which an inference is correct from the instances where it is not? The positivists, or verificationists, some of whose views are represented in this volume, are philosophers who, notwithstanding Hume's criticism of induction, propose specific criteria or conditions intended to strengthen the validity of an inductive inference. The fallibilists, or falsificationists, consider inductive inference impossible, that is, they accept Hume's criticism. Popper is the most notable falsificationist. Popper's answer to the problem of distinguishing between possibly correct and incorrect scientific statements is that real progress can be made only by attempting to disprove the statements. If you wring the rooster's neck and yet the sun rises, it follows that the rooster's crowing was not a necessary cause for the sun to rise. If a hypothesis is not disproved despite attempts to do so, it is neither proved nor disproved, but remains in conjectural limbo, subject to being disproved or modified at some later date. This view of science is one of proceeding by trial and error, or, as Popper described it, conjecture and refutation. Under this scheme there is no need for induction, which Popper dismissed as an illusion. A process of trial and error could account for my dog's behavior in learning to ring my doorbell, just as it could account for the evolution of scientific theories. The most important implication of the conjecture-and-refutation philosophy for scientific practice and thought is its focus on disproof. As Magee[5] has illustrated, one might attempt to boil a pot of water 100 or 1000 times or more, under controlled conditions, say in a laboratory in New York City, and find that each time it boils at 100°C. Even if the experiment had been repeated 1,000,000 times, however, one attempt to boil water in Denver or in a closed flask would outweigh the 1,000,000 observations and serve to refute the statement, prompting a revised and richer theory about the boiling temperature of water. The point of this argument is that the fallibilists propose that science can proceed more swiftly to discard erroneous theories and replace them with better ones by actively seeking to refute theories, rather than by fruitless accumulations of "supporting observations."

Naturally, Popper's claim that induction does not exist has tended to rile those who believe that we all use induction every day to negotiate through every aspect of our environment. The antinomy of ideas here may put them beyond synthesis, although some readers will undoubtedly wish to reconcile these opposing schools of thought enough to avoid paralysis of all inferential processes. To do so fully appears impossible, but there may be at least enough room for agreement to console the anxious reader. Certainly everyone seems to agree that empirical science does not provide irrefutable statements about nature. Inductivists believe that, *post hoc ergo propter hoc* notwithstanding, useful scientific statements can be drawn from repeated observations. Fallibilists propose that the logical role of observations is only to refute theories. For fallibilists, however, there are no restrictions on the origin of conjectural knowledge. Conjectures are not to be judged by their mode of production but only by how well they stand up to the test of experience. One way to begin reconciling the views of inductivists with those of fallibilists is to consider induction, even if nothing but a psychological illusion, to be a process that generates conjectures. Since it is legitimate for theories to derive even from dreams (and some successful ones reportedly arose from dreams), why not from induction, which even if only an illusion is at least predicated on observations? It is sometimes claimed that induction is necessary even to apply yesterday's accepted theories to today's experiences, but the process is nevertheless inescapably uncertain. For some theories, no matter how cherished, the day arrives when they no longer can be accepted. When the day comes, we need not consider the overthrow of the theory to be a logical failure of induction if we consider induction to be a road to theory formation, rather than evaluation. Of course, this view of induction sidesteps the question of whether induction can justifiably provide empirical *support* for a theory.

Some twentieth century philosophers of science, most notably Thomas Kuhn, have emphasized the role of the scientific community in determining the validity of scientific theories.[6] Critics of the fallibilist doctrine have suggested that the refutation of a theory amounts to a choice between the validity of the theory and the validity of the scientific infrastructure of theories on which the refuting observation is based. Kuhn and others have argued that the scientific community determines what is to be considered accepted and what is to be considered refuted. Kuhn's critics in turn have characterized this description of science as one of an irrational process, "a matter for mob psychology."[7] Those who cling to a belief in a rational structure for science consider Kuhn's vision to be a regrettably real description of much of what passes for scientific activity, but not prescriptive for any good science. Nevertheless, the idea that causal inference is a sociological process, whether considered descriptive or normative, is an interesting thesis that has fostered sharp debate between subjectivists and objectivists. The view that the accumulation of scientific knowledge is inherently subjective is also a tenet of the Bayesian outlook that is increasingly popular among statisticians. Subjectivism in scientific philosophy is predicated on the doctrine that the concept of truth is not merely elusive but also relative, at least in the sense that scientific truths either correspond to the beliefs of scientists or are built upon beliefs. Beliefs, of course, need not be rational and change with time, thus puncturing the concept of any objective truth. Critics of subjectivism maintain that objective knowledge exists independently of beliefs, which play no part in determining the correctness of an inference. Indeed, inference by consensus or by *ad hominem* judgment is logically fallacious because it involves belief rather than logic.

But it is not my intent here to pursue a specific philosophy of causal inference, an activity that I prefer to leave—at least on this occasion—to the contributors of this volume. With the preceding remarks I hope only to provide a simple framework to orient the reader to the discussions included here. The origin of these discussions lies in a symposium that I was asked to organize for the annual meeting of the Society for Epidemiologic Research in June, 1985. The Executive Committee of the society at first voiced some doubts about whether epidemiologists would be interested in a purely philosophical forum, but decided to give it a try. To the surprise of some, the session drew about 450 people, the largest crowd ever to attend an SER symposium, and it would have been bigger had the room been larger. Several colleagues thought that the symposium focused on issues so important to epidemiologists, and to scientists in parallel disciplines, that it should be published. I invited the four speakers to commit their contributions to paper, and I then solicited written criticisms to include as part of the published work. To complete the interchange, I asked the four primary contributors to provide rejoinders, in which they were able to address points of contention with the other speakers, reply to critics, and to clarify their original presentations.

The philosophical views presented here do not cohere, but they were not intended to present a unity of outlook. My purpose has been to focus attention on competing philosophies and how they do or might influence science. The invited participants disagree on fundamental issues, but their illuminating arguments bring the reader to the core of philosophical thinking about causal inference. For anyone who wishes to understand causal inference in scientific applications, these essays should prove invaluable.

References

1. Russell B. *The Scientific Outlook*. New York: W.W. Norton, 1931. Reprinted as "Limitations of Scientific Method" in Egner RE, Denonn LE, eds. *The Basic Writings of Bertrand Russell*. New York: Simon and Schuster, 1961:620–627.

2. Sacks HS, Berrier J, Reitman D, et al. Meta-analyses of randomized controlled trials. N Engl J Med 1987;316:450–455.

3. Relman AS. Dealing with conflicts of interest. N Engl J Med 1984;310:1182–1183.

4. Russell B. Dewey's new 'Logic.' In: Schilpp PA, ed. *The Philosophy of John Dewey.* New York: Tudor, 1939. Reprinted in Egner RE, Denonn LE, eds. *The Basic Writings of Bertrand Russell.* New York: Simon and Schuster, 1961:620–627.

5. Magee B. *Philosophy and the Real World.* La Salle, Illinois: Open Court, 1985.

6. Kuhn TS. *The Structure of Scientific Revolutions.* 2nd ed. Chicago, Illinois: University of Chicago Press, 1962.

7. Lakatos I. Falsification and the methodology of scientific research programmes. In: Lakatos I, Musgrave A, eds. *Criticism and the Growth of Knowledge.* Cambridge University Press, 1970.

THESIS

Causal Criteria and Popperian Refutation

Douglas L. Weed

Biometry Branch
National Cancer Institute
Bethesda, Maryland

It is not easy to criticize criteria.
Joseph Agassi

Nearly every epidemiologist is familiar with Hill's causal criteria[1] shown in Table 1, and many are also aware of their predecessors,[2-6] successors,[7-25] and recent examples of their implementation.[26-31] But despite this familiarity, many of these same epidemiologists would probably agree that these criteria are not totally adequate, that they provide few hard and fast rules for

Table 1. Hill's Causal Criteria

Strength of Association
Consistency
Specificity
Temporality
Biologic Gradient
Plausibility
Coherence
Experimental Evidence
Analogy

making causal inferences. To counter their shortcomings, some have advocated adding more criteria,[15] many would delete at least a few of them, and others have attempted to rank them either quantitatively[16] or qualitatively.[17]

It has also been suggested that Hill's criteria should be interpreted in terms of Popperian refutation;[32] this paper represents one response to this suggestion.

Before getting started, a few comments on the structure of this paper may be helpful. It is composed of two major sections. In the first of these, I shall get right to the heart of the matter and propose alternatives to Hill's criteria. These alternatives are based upon some basic tenets of Popperian philosophy; for example, deductive explanation. I shall not, however, review these basics, preferring instead to assume (and to hope) that most epidemiologists will have already familiarized themselves with them, and with their applications to various epidemiologic problems.[32-35]

By the end of Part One, however, it will become apparent that these new alternatives, although an improvement upon Hill's original criteria, do not fill the bill completely. To put it another way, the "Popperian" criteria do not provide a complete solution to the problem the original criteria were intended to solve, specifically, the problem of how we should go about making practical decisions about causality. Lest the reader despair, an approach to this problem is presented in Part Two of this paper. It is based upon some Popperian ideas that extend beyond the realm of scientific method.

In summary, Part One is a direct application of Popperian refutation to Hill's criteria, and Part Two provides a basis for the solution of the problem of causal decision-making in the face of scientific uncertainty.

Part One: Criticism and a Proposal

Deducing Causal Criteria from Causal Hypotheses
Given that deductive logic is an important part of an epidemiologic methodology based upon Popperian principles,[35] our first priority is to consider to what extent Hill's criteria can be de-

duced from causal hypotheses. A few examples will suffice to
show that direct deductive links between a causal hypothesis
and these familiar criteria are more often the exception than the
rule.

Example 1. Sufficient Cause

The first example is the familiar hypothesis of causal sufficiency.
It can be stated in the following manner:

If an event E (the exposure) occurs, then the event D (disease) is
always produced by it.[36]

Straightforward deductive reasoning produces the results found
in Table 2. Only two of Hill's nine original criteria—namely consistency and temporality—are directly deducible from a hypothesis of causal sufficiency. Consistency follows from this
hypothesis because for sufficient causes, the disease event is *always* produced. Temporality is also an integral part of such a
causal hypothesis, as Rothman[20] has suggested. (It is interesting
to point out that, in general terms, causality need not require
antecedence. Counterexamples include simultaneous cause-effect
relationships, and in theoretical physics—where time can have
peculiar habits—effects may actually precede causes.[37] In an attempt to include all of these possibilities, Bunge has suggested
that causes have an "existential priority" over their effects.)

Table 2. Hill's Criteria and Causal Sufficiency

Directly deducible	Consistency
	Temporality
Not deducible (unless hypothesis is altered)	Preventability ("experimental evidence")
	Strength of association
	Specificity
	Biologic gradient
Not deducible	Plausibility
	Coherence
	Analogy

Four other criteria—preventability (what Hill called "experimental evidence"), strength of association, specificity, and biologic gradient—are not directly deducible from this hypothesis. These will be considered in turn.

At first glance, it seems reasonable to assert that preventability follows from causal sufficiency, because if the exposure is removed, then the disease event that is always produced by this exposure when it is present would not now occur.

This is not quite the case, however, because causal sufficiency does not preclude other causes from acting, causes that may themselves produce a similar disease event. Therefore, only if an additional constraint is included—namely that no other sufficient cause acts—will the deductive link between this causal hypothesis and preventability be assured. Unfortunately, the addition of this constraint creates a new hypothesis, and it is not one of causal sufficiency. Rather, it is the hypothesis of causal necessity in which an event occurs *if and only if* the cause occurs.

Similar arguments apply to the criterion of the strength of an association. Deducing a large ("strong") value for an effect measure also depends upon what is hypothesized about the presence of other causes.[38] This fact is illustrated in Figure 1. Because causal sufficiency can be equivalently written as

If E, then not-D is impossible,

we can represent causal sufficiency in a simple 2 x 2 table with a zero in the $(E,\bar{D})$ cell.[32] Computational formulas for the relative risk (RR) and risk difference (RD) reveal that the magnitude of the effect is dependent upon the risk in the "unexposed" and therefore upon the presence of other causes.

The remaining two criteria that are also not directly deducible from the hypothesis of causal sufficiency (without alterations in that hypothesis) are specificity and biologic gradient. The reasons for this are straightforward: specificity requires causal necessity, while biologic gradient, or dose-response,[18] is not deduced because a sufficient cause produces an all-or-none response.

Three of Hill's original criteria remain to be considered: plausi-

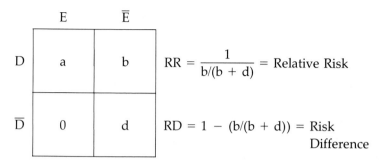

Figure 1
2 × 2 Table for Causal Sufficiency and resultant Effect Measures

bility, coherence, and analogy. Like most of the others already encountered, these three are not deducible from a hypothesis of causal sufficiency. Unlike the others, however, we can go further and say that these three are not deducible from *any* hypothesis.

For example, consider both plausibility and coherency. (Some previous commentators[7,10,15] have also collapsed the criteria of plausibility and coherency into one. Others, most notably Sackett,[14] have suggested substituting "epidemiologic sense" and biologic sense" for plausibility and coherency.) It makes little sense to say that, given a particular hypothesis, we can deduce its plausibility or coherency. On the other hand, it makes good sense to say that either one or both of these criteria suggest the act of deduction itself. In other words, if an association is deducible from some causal hypothesis, then it is reasonable to conclude that the hypothesis is a plausible one. Coherency, in a similar manner, is also related to the extent to which some hypothesis fits into a theoretical framework.

Analogy, on the other hand, has little to do with deductive logic at all. Hill[1] used the criterion of analogy to give credibility to an untested hypothesis that is similar in some way to another tested and corroborated hypothesis. For example, if we consider the hypothesis that drug A causes disease D_1 and we "know" that drug B causes disease D_2 (similar to disease D_1), then the hypothesis that A causes D_1 is strengthened. But this use of analogy has more to do with an inductive (verificationist) methodology than with a deductive (refutationist) methodology, and therefore must be revised. Although it may be tempting to suggest that a hypothesis is supported by the fact that similar hypotheses have been verified elsewhere (for example, in other species), *analogy best describes one source of untested hypotheses.* And according to Popperian principles, how an epidemiologist goes about inventing hypotheses is decidedly not a logical process.[35,39]

Example 2. Component Cause

The second example involves the hypothesis that a number of component causes constitute a sufficient cause.[40] A cursory glance is all that is required to convince oneself that deducing causal criteria from the hypothesis of a component cause is even less rewarding than it was in this previous example of a sufficient cause. Only temporality remains as a directly deducible criterion, while consistency joins the ranks of those criteria "not deducible, unless the hypothesis is altered." Finally, the above remarks about the criteria of plausibility, coherence, and analogy again hold true. These results are summarized in Table 3.

Example 3. A Cause Acting in a Multistage Disease Process

The third example involves causes that act within a theory for a disease process. Consider the multistage theory of carcinogenesis in which external causes (or carcinogens) alter the rates at which

Table 3. Hill's Criteria and a Component Cause

Directly deducible	Temporality
Not deducible (unless hypothesis is altered)	Consistency Preventability Strength of association Specificity Biologic gradient
Not deducible	Plausibility Coherence Analogy

cancer occurs.[41] In contrast to the first two examples above, the multistage theory explicitly incorporates other, background causes within its structure. This permits more precise and detailed deductions. Specifically, it is possible to deduce the strength of the association, consistency, temporality, preventability, and biologic gradient.[42,43] Specificity, plausibility, coherence, and analogy remain as before—not deducible. These results are summarized in Table 4.

A Popperian Alternative to Hill's Criteria

The examples above reveal the first Popperian alternative to Hill's criteria: *predictability*. It means that once a causal hypothesis has been proposed, it is then possible to deduce from it certain predictions, in preparation for comparing them with empirical observations. Note that this criterion is not dependent upon the particular form of the causal hypothesis. As shown above, each example revealed important differences, yet the basic methodology was always the same; namely, propose a hypothesis and deduce predictions from it.

It is important to point out that the criterion of predictability is equally applicable to noncausal hypotheses that purport to explain other phenomena of interest to epidemiologists. A recent example involves the effect of selection on mortality rates in occupational populations.[34]

Although predictability is a necessary part of a Popperian ap-

Table 4. Hill's Criteria and the Multistage Model

Directly deducible	Strength of association
	Consistency
	Temporality
	Preventability
	Biologic gradient
Not deducible	Specificity
	Plausibility
	Coherence
	Analogy

proach to causal inference, it alone is not sufficient. We must also take care to assure ourselves that hypotheses are *testable*, that their predicted consequences are capable of conflicting with observations and that we have done all that we can to improve the opportunity for those conflicts. An important strategy for improving the testability of a hypothesis is to increase the precision of its predictions. More precise predictions explicitly reveal not only which observations are compatible with the hypothesis but also which observations are incompatible with the hypothesis, i.e., which observations test the hypothesis. In sum, *testability* becomes our second new criterion.

Except for the criterion of analogy, all of Hill's original criteria are subsumed under the two criteria proposed above. Predictability, or the process whereby observable characteristics are deduced from causal hypotheses, begets what might reasonably be called Hill's "hypothesis dependent" criteria of consistency, strength, dose-response, temporality, preventability, and specificity. These are called "hypothesis dependent" because, as demonstrated above, they may differ, depending upon the particular hypothesis under consideration. Testability, in turn, lays down a potent condition upon the predictions deduced from that hypothesis; they must not be so vague that any conceivable observation will confirm them.

One of Hill's original criteria remains to be considered. Analogy, in Popperian terms, does not relate to the methodological practice of deducing predictions from causal hypotheses nor of testing these predictions against observations. Rather, it relates to the origin of hypotheses, and so to how we as scientists "come-up-with-them" in the first place. Analogy, then, becomes one way to invent a hypothesis, although it is a bit unimaginative. A Popperian alternative to analogy would be: creative inventiveness.

In summary, *the Popperian alternatives to Hill's causal criteria are quite simply: predictability and testability* (see Table 5). Excluding analogy, these general criteria for epidemiologic inference not only fully subsume Hill's original criteria, but as importantly, they also permit the emergence of new (hypothesis dependent)

**Table 5. General Criteria for
Epidemiological Inference**

Predictability
Testability

criteria. One example would be the predictions about the age
dependency of cancer incidence from theories such as the multistage model of carcinogenesis and from assumptions about the
position (i.e., early/late) of the purported carcinogen in this disease process. Another example would be predictions about the
age dependency of mortality rate differences in studies of the
"healthy worker effect."

Despite such favorable features, these general criteria of predictability and testability will not solve all the problems pertinent
to a comprehensive treatment of epidemiologic inference. To put
it more precisely, they only provide a solution to one of three
fundamental causal problems in epidemiology. These three problems are the focus of Part Two.

Part Two: Problems and More on Criticism

Three Problems of Cause
Undoubtedly there is a whole range of problems important to
the rather broad issue of epidemiologic inference but, for my
purposes here, three merit close attention. In general terms,
these are:

1) the *ontologic* problem of cause

2) the *methodological* (or epistemologic) problem of cause and

3) the *ethical* problem of cause.

The ontologic problem has to do with the nature or form of
causal hypotheses. Its solution must include answers to questions such as: What are causal hypotheses? What is their relation
to (i.e., how do they differ from) other kinds of hypotheses? Are
there causal laws and causal ranges of laws?[44]

In Part One of this paper, three distinctly different causal hypotheses were considered: causal sufficiency, a component of sufficient cause, and a cause that acts within the construct of a general explanation for a disease process. Undoubtedly there are others, for example, more than one "interdependent" cause,[45] or both causes and preventives acting in concert[46] as well as within the construct of a general disease theory.[47] It is noteworthy that the inclusion of cause within a more general explanation is consistent with Popper's view on this matter.[48]

The second (methodological) problem of cause primarily involves the ways in which we go about gaining knowledge about cause from our observations. It, like the ontologic problem, can also be examined by attempting answers to questions, but these, of course, are somewhat different. Examples are: What are the observable characteristics of causal hypotheses? How do we test causal hypotheses? How do we gain theoretical knowledge about cause from our observations?

In Part One, much of the ink was devoted to illustrating the important fact that the initial choice of a causal hypothesis (i.e., one's tentative solution to the ontologic problem of cause) will determine which observable characteristics are predicted (i.e., deduced), and therefore which criteria could be used in testing that hypothesis. Indeed, although one can consider the ontologic problem as distinct from the methodological problem, it is clear that they are closely linked. Simply put, you can't attempt to test a hypothesis without first stating it.

One may reasonably conclude then that the "Popperian" criteria, namely predictability and testability, (along with a healthy dose of creative inventiveness) provide epidemiologists with an explicit (and in other sciences, a widely recognized) solution to the problem of gaining theoretical knowledge from experience.[49] But this methodological problem is clearly not the only one that Hill and others set out to solve. Undoubtedly they also wanted a solution to the ethical problem of cause, which like the others has its attendant questions, such as: "How shall we choose the right hypothesis to act upon?" and, "When is it appropriate to act, given our more or less uncertain knowledge of cause?"

It is the purpose of the remainder of this section to examine how Popper's solution to the problem of gaining (causal) knowledge from experience suggests a solution to the problem of causal action.

One reason why a solution to the problem of causal decision-making depends upon the solutions to the problems of causal ontology and causal methodology is that it is unreasonable to countenance such decisions without some research—in the form of hypothesis-testing—preceding them. We could, of course, hold the contrary opinion that decisions could be made on the basis of observations alone. But this idea does not hold up under close scrutiny; all observations are theory laden; all observations are undertaken with some preconceived hypothesis in mind. (This concept has been previously discussed in epidemiologic terms;[32,35] another good example of it can be found in a recent debate over the choice of subjects in case-control/referent studies.[50,51] There it is quite clear that one's hypothesis determines to a great extent which set of "controls" is appropriate to test that hypothesis.) It follows that even those observations that jump out at us, that we claim are "unexpected," only attract our attention because they failed to match some, perhaps hazy, expectation for them.

This link between the first two problems and the third also results in the following difficulty: the solutions to the first two problems—namely that the forms of hypotheses are infinitely varied and that these hypotheses are *always* subject to failure (indeed, the more testable they are, the better they are)—results in a healthy dose of uncertainty. The scientific process never ends up with certain knowledge about cause nor about explanations within which causes may produce these effects. All hypotheses are always in a state of potential change, and we are always faced with the possibility that we will be surprised by what we discover.

How then can we make reasonable decisions to act, in the face of this certain uncertainty?

Of course, it will be impossible to discuss all that should be considered regarding such decisions, primarily because in the end these decisions usually involve such issues as economics (and therefore politics). Because these are somewhat beyond the scope of this paper, I will instead focus upon a general (philosophical) approach to decision making.

Alternatives to Certainty

Given that certainty is impossible, there are at least three alternatives to consider: belief, probability, and criticism. (For example, "Among those who have examined the aspects of an observed association that lead us *to believe* it is causal is Sir A.B. Hill";[20] "What aspects of an association should we especially consider before deciding that the *most likely* interpretation of it is causation?"[1] (emphasis added); see Settle[49] for a discussion of criticism.)

Some of the difficulties with using belief in cause as a basis for epidemiologic inference have already been discussed.[35] In brief, belief in a particular cause may prevent us from making sincere attempts to test it as strenuously as possible. Furthermore, belief in causal explanation as *the only* form of explanation (to the exclusion of others) may lead to a stagnation of scientific progress in epidemiology.

More generally, the problem with belief as a basis for making decisions about causality is that it makes it somewhat easier to conceal error. Some of the best illustrations of this fact can be found outside science, in the realm of religion. There, a belief in some deity or creed often results in a total cessation of critical inquiry, or what has been appropriately called a "retreat to commitment." Parallels to scientific inquiry, although sometimes amusing,[52] are not at all far-fetched.[53,54]

Although popular with some, the use of probability as an alternative to certainty has its own lion's share of problems. Decision procedures that allow us to assign probabilities to hypotheses given evidence do not usually prescribe whether more evidence should be obtained, nor do they help us to determine whether some existing evidence should be ignored.[49] Although probability may be reasonably incorporated into our ontologic battery (e.g., as the random alternative to causality) it seems less reasonable to assign arbitrary probabilistic values or "scores" to our findings, tally them up, and act accordingly.

The third alternative to certainty is critical debate or simply, criticism. The importance of criticism as a solution to the third problem of cause—the problem of causal action—can best be shown by first discussing its role in the solution to the second (methodologic) problem of cause. As scientists, we shall often begin our inquiries with an observation that fails to agree with our prediction for it. For example, if a prediction is based upon chance and our observation fails to agree with that prediction, then we say that our observation is "statistically significant." But we don't stop here; we proceed by proposing other solutions to the same problem, which take the form of alternative explanations. Examples of these include cause (in its variety of guises), other noncausal theories, confounders, bias, etc. We then try to eliminate errors in these tentative alternatives by *criticizing* them, which means that we deduce predictions from them and test these against the original or (better yet) more precise observations. Ensuing conflicts, as might be expected, lead us to new problems. In the end, the cycle of problem definition, tentative solutions, and criticism repeats itself.

In a manner similar to that described for hypotheses, our decisions to act should also be criticized in the hopes of improving them. For example, we can propose interventions and critically examine their implications in terms of risks and benefits. We can then make corrective changes as a result of this criticism, whether in the intervention itself or in the manner in which it is administered.

The value of criticism lies in its ability to bring weaknesses to the surface. These weaknesses are to be found in our public-health actions, just as they are to be found in the hypotheses from which they arise. And, although such criticism will never make us certain, it will help us to avoid being more wrong than we need to be.

Conclusion

Criticism is not only a reasonable philosophical guide to epidemiologic inference and to public health action, it is also the theme that runs through this paper, although this theme remains somewhat understated. Recall however, that in Part One I criticized Hill's criteria, thus paving the way for some more general alternatives. In Part Two, I criticized these new criteria in terms of their usefulness as guides to practical action. So it goes: a problem is introduced, its proposed solutions in turn are criticized. New problems and new solutions are then bound to emerge, and all the while progress is apparent.

As a final critical note, I should briefly discuss my choice of the introductory quote by Joseph Agassi.[55] The reason why it isn't easy to criticize criteria is that you must first convince those who depend upon them that there is room for improvement. As Agassi suggests, one way to accomplish this Herculean task is to simply come up with a "barrage of diverse counterexamples" as I have attempted in the first section of this paper. Fortunately or unfortunately, (depending on your point of view) my so-called counterexamples were not complete in their devastation. It is unquestionably true that some of Hill's original criteria will continue to provide epidemiologists with a basis for inference. But I cannot overemphasize the fact that the value of any of these survivors is largely dependent upon the particular hypothesis to be tested. In sum, from different hypotheses come different predictions.

In conclusion, general criteria for epidemiologic inference are proposed: namely, *predictability* and *testability*. These are not simply substitutes for the familiar causal criteria. Rather, they explain earlier criteria and, as importantly, they also improve upon them by providing the methodologic framework for new hypothesis-dependent criteria. Therefore, these general criteria must represent progress in our methodological knowledge, because a better method will both explain and correct earlier methods.[56,57]

Acknowledgments

I would like to thank my colleague, Bruce Trock, for his helpful suggestions, and Carol Ball, for help in preparing the manuscript.

References

1. Hill AB. The environment and disease: association or causation? Proc Roy Soc Med 1965;58:295–300.

2. Yerushalmy J, Palmer CE. On the methodology of investigations of etiologic factors in chronic diseases. J Chronic Dis 1959;10:27–40.

3. Lilienfeld AM. "On the methodology of investigations of etiologic factors in chronic diseases." Some comments. J Chronic Dis 1959;10:41–46.

4. Sartwell PE. "On the methodology of investigations of etiologic factors in chronic diseases." Further comments. J Chronic Dis 1960;11:61–63.

5. Surgeon General's Advisory Committee on Smoking and Health. *Smoking and Health 1964.* Rockville, Maryland: Public Health Service; DHEW publication no. (PHS)1103.

6. Bollet AJ. On seeking the cause of disease. Clin Res 1964;12:305–310.

7. Wynder EL. The Identification of Causal Factors in Noncommunicable Diseases by Statistical Means. In: Ingelfinger FJ, et al., eds. *Controversy in Internal Medicine.* Philadelphia: Saunders, 1966;2:649–658.

8. Yerushalmy J. On inferring causality from observed associations. In: Ingelfinger FJ, et al., eds. *Controversy in Internal Medicine.* Philadelphia: Saunders, 1966;2:659–668.

9. Susser M. Criteria of judgment. In: *Causal Thinking in the Health Sciences: Concepts and Strategies in Epidemiology.* New York: Oxford Univ, 1973:140–162.

10. MacMahon B, Pugh TF. Concepts of cause. In: *Epidemiology: Principles and Methods.* Boston: Little, Brown, 1974:17–27.

11. Evans AS. Causation and disease: the Henle-Koch postulates revisited. Yale J Biol Med 1976;49:175–195.

12. Susser M. Judgment and causal inference: criteria in epidemiologic studies. Am J Epidemiol 1977;105:1–15.

13. Evans AS. Causation and disease: a chronological journey. Am J Epidemiol 1978;108:249–258.

14. Sackett DL. The diagnosis of causation. In: Gent M, Shigematsu I, eds. *Epidemiological Issues in Reported Drug-induced Illnesses—S.M.O.N. and Other Examples.* Hamilton, Ontario: McMaster Univ Lib Press, 1978:106–117.

15. Feinstein AR. Scientific standards vs. statistical associations and biologic logic in the analysis of causation. Clin Pharmacol Ther 1979;25: 481–492.

16. Dinman BD, Sussman NB. Uncertainty, risk, and the role of epidemiology in public policy development. J Occup Med 1983;25:511–516.

17. Feinstein AR. Efficacy of different research structures in preventing bias in the analysis of causation. Clin Pharmacol Ther 1979;26:129–141.

18. Weiss NS. Inferring causal relationships: elaboration of the criterion of "dose-response." Am J Epidemiol 1981;113:487–490.

19. Kleinbaum DG, Kupper LL, Morgenstern H. Fundamentals of epidemiologic research. In: *Epidemiologic Research*. Belmont, California: Lifetime Learning, 1982:19–39.

20. Rothman KJ. Causation and causal inference. In: Schottenfeld D, Fraumeni J, eds. *Cancer Epidemiology and Prevention*. Philadelphia: Saunders, 1982:15–22.

21. U.S. Department of Health and Human Services. Epidemiologic criteria for causality. In: *The Health Consequences of Smoking: Cancer*. Rockville, Maryland: Public Health Service. Publication. no. (PHS)82-50179, 1982;16–20.

22. Lower GM, Kanarek MS. Conceptual/operational criteria of causality: relevance to systematic epidemiologic theory. Med Hypoth 1983;11:217–244.

23. Burch PRJ. The Surgeon General's "Epidemiologic criteria for causality." A critique. J Chronic Dis 1983;36:821–836.

24. Lilienfeld AM. The Surgeon General's "Epidemiologic criteria for causality." A criticism of Burch's critique. J Chronic Dis 1983;36:837–845.

25. Burch, PRJ. The Surgeon General's "Epidemiologic criteria for causality." Reply to Lilienfeld [Letter]. J Chronic Dis 1984;37:148–156.

26. Cabelli VJ, Dufour AP, McCabe LJ, Levin MA. Swimming-associated gastroenteritis and water quality. Am J Epidemiol 1982;115:606–616.

27. Broadhead WE, Kaplan BH, James SA, et al. The epidemiologic evidence for a relationship between social support and health. Am J Epidemiol 1983;117:521–537.

28. Rohan TE. Alcohol and ischemic heart disease: a review. Aust NZ J Med 1984;14:75–80.

29. Arthur MJP, Hall AJ, Wright R. Hepatitis B, hepatocellular carcinoma, and strategies for prevention. Lancet 1984;1(8377):607–610.

30. Cates W. Sexually transmitted organisms and infertility: the proof of the pudding. Sex Transm Dis 1984;11:113–116.

31. Daniels SR, Greenberg RS, Ibrahim MA. Scientific uncertainties in the studies of salicylate use and Reye's syndrome. JAMA 1983;249:1311–1316.

32. Maclure M. Popperian refutation in epidemiology. Am J Epidemiol 1985;121:343–350.

33. Buck C. Popper's philosophy for epidemiologists. Int J Epidemiol 1975;4:159–168.

34. Weed, DL. An epidemiological application of Popper's method. J Epidemiol Community Health 1985;39:277–285.

35. Weed DL. On the logic of causal inference. Am J Epidemiol 1986;123:965–979.

36. Bunge M. Formulations of the causal principle. In: *Causality and Modern Science*. 3rd ed. New York: Dover, 1979:31–53.

37. Bunge M. An examination of the empiricist critique of causality. In: *Causality and Modern Science*. 3rd ed. New York: Dover, 1979:57–88.

38. Weed DL, Trock B. Criticism and the growth of epidemiologic knowledge [Letter]. Am J Epidemiol 1986;123:1119–1120.

39. Popper KR. Elimination of psychologism. In: *The Logic of Scientific Discovery*. Revised ed. New York: Harper and Row, 1968:31–32. Originally published as *Logik der Forschung*. Vienna: Springer, 1934.

40. Rothman KJ. Causes. Am J Epidemiol 1976;104:587–592.

41. Peto J. In mouse skin and in man. In: Borzsonyi M, Day NE, et al., eds. *Models, Mechanisms and Aetiology of Tumour Promotion*. IARC Sci Publ 1985;56:359–373.

42. Day NE, Brown CC. Multistage models and primary prevention of cancer. J Natl Cancer Inst 1980;64:977–989.

43. Moolgavkar SH, Knudson AG. Mutation and cancer: a model for human carcinogenesis. J Natl Cancer Inst 1981;66:1037–1052.

44. Bunge M. Preface to the Dover Edition. In: *Causality and Modern Science*. 3rd ed. New York: Dover, 1979:xv–xxii.

45. Miettinen OS. Causal and preventive interdependence: elementary principles. Scand J Work Environ Health 1982;8:159–168.

46. Dayal HH. Additive excess risk model for epidemiologic interaction in retrospective studies. J Chronic Dis 1980;33:653–660.

47. Trock B, Weed D. Predicting the effects of retinoid chemoprevention [Abstract]. Am J Epidemiol 1985;122:521–522.

48. Popper KR. The bucket and the searchlight: two theories of knowledge. Appendix 1 of: *Objective Knowledge: An Evolutionary Approach*. Oxford University Press, 1979:341–361.

49. Settle T. Induction and Probability Unfused. In: Schilpp PA, ed. *The Philosophy of Karl Popper*. Library of Living Philosophers. Vol. XIV, Book II. La Salle, Illinois: Open Court, 1974:697–749.

50. Miettinen OS. The "case-control" study: valid selection of subjects. J Chronic Dis 1985;38:543–548.

51. Schlesselman JJ. Valid selection of subjects in case-control studies. J Chronic Dis 1985;38:549–550.

52. Rimm AA, Bortin M. Clinical trials as a religion. Biomedicine 1978;28(special issue):60–63.

53. Weaver W. A Scientist Ponders Faith. Saturday Review 1959 Jan 3:8–10, 33.

54. Bartley WW. *The Retreat to Commitment*. 2nd ed. La Salle: Open Court, 1984.

55. Agassi J. On Novelty. In: Cohen RD, Wartofsky MW, eds. *Science in Flux. Boston Studies in the Philosophy of Science.* Dordrecht: D. Reidel, 1975:28:51–73.

56. Popper KR. The aim of science. In: *Objective Knowledge: An Evolutionary Approach.* Oxford University Press, 1979:191–205.

57. Bartley WW. Appendix 2. Logical strength and demarcation. In: *The Retreat to Commitment.* 2nd ed. La Salle: Open Court, 1984:185–209.

Falsification, Verification and Causal Inference in Epidemiology: Reconsiderations in the Light of Sir Karl Popper's Philosophy*

Mervyn Susser

Gertrude H. Sergievsky Center
Columbia University

Paradigms, Deduction and Induction

In epidemiology, judgments about causality must defer to a torrent of new knowledge. The evidence to hand changes from year to year, and even from month to month. Kuhn's[1] thesis of scientific revolution may be taken to dispute this point about change. He has argued forcefully that the evidence normally drawn on by scientists is dictated by an overriding contemporary paradigm—a term Kuhn uses variously, but in this sense to describe the guiding theoretical concepts of a science. The paradigm will shape the way in which any given generation of scientists construes a causal sequence. Revolutionary change, relatively infrequent, accompanies paradigm change; thereafter some parts of previous knowledge and previous ideas become irrelevant to the new focus.

To illustrate changes in paradigm, the example of tuberculosis will serve. Rudolph Virchow, the leading pathologist of mid-nineteenth century Germany, described tuberculosis in a celebrated phrase as "a social disease." Later, once Robert Koch in

* This paper also appears in *Epidemiology, Health and Society: Selected Essays*, Susser M. New York: Oxford University Press, 1987.

the 1880's had discovered the tubercle bacillus and its role in disease, the causal attribution switched to the bacillus. A new paradigm, the germ theory, governed a notion of causality that attributed specific diseases to specific agents. A variety of manifestations of what had been called phthisis were shed and assigned to other diseases; only the pathologies that kept company with the new bacillus were retained for tuberculosis or reassigned to it.[2] Pathology was tailored to fit the tubercle bacillus as the single and specific cause of tuberculosis, in a way that made it rationally coherent with the new paradigm of the germ theory.

In our day, the paradigm of the germ theory too has fallen by the wayside. We adhere to a theory of multiple causes: to the tubercle bacillus as agent, any present-day epidemiologist would add a bundle of causes such as family exposure, genetic susceptibility, poor nutrition, and overcrowding.

Most of the time, contention on the revolutionary scale of a paradigm change is not an issue in epidemiology. The criteria for causal inference—which in truth are no more than guideposts for judgment—can generally be applied under the umbrella of a single paradigm. Nonetheless, change retains a central place for an epidemiologist who would apply criteria for attributing causality. Cause is established in a continuing and evolving process. Criteria embody the values we implicitly choose to attach to the properties of our observations. Some of the criteria themselves depend on the evolution of the processes that lead us to conclusions about causality. Thus to attribute cause at any point in time is to take a snapshot. A well-based conclusion is produced only by the unfolding of a continuing serial with a theme carried this way and that in constant replication.

Hence, a single study is seldom if ever conclusive. Four centuries ago Francis Bacon had understood the nature of causal inference as a process of exclusions and affirmations. He wrote:

The induction which is to be available for the discovery and the demonstration of sciences and arts, must analyze nature by proper rejections and exclusions; and then after a sufficient number of negatives, come to a conclusion on the affirmative instances.[3]

Note that Bacon describes induction, a process that moves from the particular to the general. In this respect, the process does not fit the prescription of Sir Karl Popper, one of the most influential philosophers of science of the 20th century who, after an introduction by Carol Buck,[4] has recently and somewhat late become fashionable in epidemiology.

Popper argues that science advances by the process of deduction alone.[5] We begin with a hypothesis—an act of invention and imagination—and can reach a conclusion only to the extent that the hypothesis can be rejected. In this regard, Popper is in accord with Bacon's "rejections and exclusions." However, Popper allows no room in the scientific process for verification, and none for induction, which is entirely to abandon the use of the "affirmatives" recommended by Bacon. For Popper, induction is not a logical but a psychological process. One can never know all the particular facts that would ensure the validity of a generalization: in Popper's example, to assert from innumerable observations that all swans are white does not protect the affirmation against the later discovery of a non-white swan.

In one central aspect of Popper's philosophy many epidemiologists will concur. He demarcates a scientific from a non-scientific theory by its testability (in theoretical and not necessarily in immediate practical terms). It follows that the theories and hypotheses likely to produce the most secure knowledge are the most testable, and the most testable are the most falsifiable. Ideally such theories have universality (i.e., cover a wide range of conditions), simplicity (involve the least number of assumptions, qualifications, auxiliary hypotheses, or parameters) and precision. They are formulated *a priori* as predictions, and tested against a system of "basic statements" (existing singular facts). These characteristics put them at maximum risk of falsification.

A second central aspect of Popper's philosophy is that "falsification" and "corroboration" are asymmetrical. The asymmetry follows from his dismissal of induction and verification. Falsification on testing allows a hypothesis to be rejected; failure to falsify does not affirm, but merely "corroborates," in that the theory survives. The degree to which a theory is corroborated depends on the number of tests it has survived, and more particularly on the severity of the tests in terms of universality, simplicity and precision. However severe the tests, survival of a theory is provisional and does not verify it.

In accord with Popper, epidemiologists commonly do assign the highest criterion value to tests of hypotheses that are *a priori*, simple, and falsifiable. In at least two important aspects, however, I depart from Popper's position. The first aspect is in the supposed asymmetry between falsification and "corroboration" which, in practice, I do not find to be nearly as extreme as Popper holds it to be. Falsification is undoubtedly a critical element in the advance of knowledge. It follows from Popper's preference for testing those hypotheses that are most falsifiable that he also prefers those that are least probable. The choice of improbable hypotheses will not recommend itself to epidemiologists who may have to undertake large-scale studies spanning many years. With more promising hypotheses, the high risk procedure of disproof by deduction is not less fallible than is that of verification of proof; in any single test both kinds of result are ultimately provisional.

The second aspect of my disagreement is in the matter of induction: to rule out induction as well as verification is to rule out much of the rational (and non-rational) procedure of day-to-day science, and to deprive the scientist of his small arms if not his biggest guns. Certainly epidemiologists are in the habit of generating hypotheses by induction from the arrays of descriptive data and existing knowledge with which their studies are bound to begin. Every probability statement about a sample population must be extrapolated by induction to become a general statement.

In short, even if Popper's arguments were entirely sound (and several philosophers do not agree that they are), he offers an ideal model. This model is founded on logic and exemplified in the main from physics; it is not a working model founded on the realities of the epidemiologic enterprise. Of necessity scientists are pragmatists. When they must ignore philosophers they do, and they proceed with the business of verification and of induction as well as with more formal attempts at falsification by deduction.

The central concern of causal inference is to establish preference among theories at a given point in time. In making such decisions, we cannot do without induction. At any given time, indeed, no test of a deduction from a theory may be available. So I shall follow Bacon in using both "exclusions" and "affirmations," and both induction and deduction, in the process of causal inference.

Properties of Causes

The pragmatic concept of a cause or determinant is any factor that makes a difference: in a given situation it has an effect or brings about change. In epidemiology, we recognize the possible presence of a cause of a health disorder in a population by its coincidence, outside agreed bounds of chance, with the supposed effect. That is to say, the suspect factor (X) and the outcome (Y) are statistically associated. The probability that an association exists is the first criterion commonly deployed in causal inference in epidemiology.

Two properties inhere in the relations of cause and effect.[6] Both must be present in any association that has a claim to be causal. One is the property of *time-order* (that is, X precedes Y). The other is the property of *direction* (that is, X leads to Y).

That a cause must precede its effect seems obvious. To demonstrate the fact, however, is often not simple. Time order is most readily shown in experiment. X can be added or removed at a known time and ensuing change observed. But in some other kinds of design, the order of the variables in time is seen "as through a glass darkly." I shall give the property of time order a place to itself as a criterion.

Direction implies an asymmetrical relation between a supposed cause and effect. There is no asymmetry in the fact that day follows night; the movement of the earth causes both. Direction, too, is most readily seen with interventions—something added or removed—as in the results of randomized experiment. Even flawless experiment is but one piece in an assembly of evidence about causality, however, and not enough in itself. To infer that a factor does indeed produce a supposed effect, several criteria need to be deployed. Thus I shall address five criteria that bear on the existence of the property of direction in an association. These are strength, consistency, specificity, predictive performance and coherence.

Throughout the following discussion, I make the unrealistic assumption that the design and execution of all studies is unexceptionable. Design and execution may strengthen or undermine the assembly of data on which inference draws. For example, well-executed experimental interventions narrow the scope for uncertainty left by observational studies, but at the cost of generalizability. The criteria by which designs are assessed, however, are different from criteria for inference. (Some authors include research method as a criterion for inference, and give special weight to experiment.[7] While design must be taken into account in the overall judgment of a study, I do not consider it to be an attribute of an *association*.) Studies must be scrutinized for the quality of the measurement of all variables included.

In addition, studies must be closely screened for confounding, which may arise from a multitude of potential biases, and artifactually either enhance or suppress associations. Finally, analytic elaboration is essential not only to rooting out confounding but to deriving a valid estimate of the unique contribution of a hypothetical causal variable to an observed association.

The procedures of screening for confounding and of elaboration, like those of design and execution, pose a study in themselves.[6] I shall here confine discussion to criteria for causal inference. In this treatment I introduce probability as a criterion of judgment, whereas previously I have treated it separately (as a means of quantifying and excluding chance events); and I add predictive performance as yet another criterion. Questions of falsification (or rejection) and verification (or affirmation) receive particular attention.

The criteria to be discussed are mutually supportive rather than mutually exclusive; they are not hard and fast categories, but overlapping and complementary. Only some criteria on some occasions can be decisive. Rejection of an hypothesis can be accomplished with confidence by only three criteria (time order, consistency, and factual incompatibility or incoherence) and strong affirmation by only four (strength, consistency, predictive performance and statistical coherence in the form of a regular exposure/effect relation). In many instances, we can argue only that the criterion supports or detracts from a causal judgment.

I. Probability

Probabilities serve to set limits for decisions about whether an association between two variables exists. The decisions rest on estimates of whether the association falls outside the bounds of the variation to be expected for the universe under study. These probabilities have no bearing on either the time order or the direction of the variables involved. On their own, they serve chiefly to guide interest in further exploration.

To apply probabilities to experimental and observational studies, a consensus has evolved about a set of conventions that rule the procedures of statistical inference. These conventions for hypothesis testing accord well with Popper's requirements for the falsification of *a priori* hypotheses. A hypothesis must be clearly formulated before testing, and the aim is to reject the null hypothesis of no difference. What is at odds with Popper is the affirmative character assigned by most to a significant result.

The procedures that allow us to so conclude about the meaning of a statistical test cannot be completed if, with Popper, we outlaw induction. The statement of probabilities, we have noted, requires induction about the relations of a sample to the universe from which it is drawn.[8] The level of statistical significance is such a statement about the frequency with which a finding is likely to arise by chance. This criterion has great currency in the world of medicine today. A study in which conventionally set levels of statistical significance are not met is likely to be given short shrift.

Failure to satisfy the quantitative criterion of statistical significance does indeed help in deciding how much attention to give a particular result. The criterion is less decisive than it is often made to appear, however. The presence of statistical significance is grounds for rejecting the formal statistical (null) hypothesis of no association posed by a particular study, and for inferring that the association is unlikely to be owed to chance. Conversely, lack of statistical significance on its own is grounds for inferring that an association has some preset probability of being owed to chance (that is, the null hypothesis cannot be rejected).

Lack of significance gives quantitative but not logical grounds for rejecting an epidemiologic hypothesis. The weight attached to statistical significance probably contributes to a bias towards skepticism that I believe can be detected in the judgmental procedures of epidemiology. At the least it is necessary to bring to bear, in addition, the criterion of statistical power. With small populations at risk, this estimate may show that a moderate effect has little chance if any of being detected.

The question of statistical testing is by no means straightforward, and a sound assessment of statistical significance is complex. Indeed, many epidemiologists in these days generally prefer to use a different statistic—namely, confidence limits—to weigh the probabilities of a chance finding. Confidence limits indicate the values within which a given proportion (say 90 or 95 per cent) of all findings are likely to fall.

This more informative statistic does not reduce the complexity of the issues. Virtually always, in contemporary epidemiology, many variables are under consideration at once. Relations that are a factorial of that number can be examined in any single analysis. In addition, many variables may interact with each other and thereby modify their relations with still other variables. Only some of these relations will have been proposed as hypotheses *a priori*. The "dredging of data" and the resulting construction of hypotheses after the fact—that is, exploration of data to seek out and test relations between variables not explicitly stated beforehand—does not carry the same logical weight as the test of an hypothesis formulated before the test. The probabilities of finding significant results are raised by such procedures. Threshold levels attached by convention to the formal hypothesis test therefore need to be raised, but the procedures in use are mostly unsatisfying.

One may sum up the issue of statistical inference by saying that if the criterion of statistical significance is not met and power is adequate, one may count the test on the side of falsification. If the criterion of significance is not met but power is lacking, the test is not null, but indeterminate. If the criterion of significance is met—whether or not power is adequate—then the result is outside the preset bound of chance and affirmative. In statistical inference, consensual conventions are applied to quantify probabilities. The limits set are arbitrary, and do not override logical inference based on other criteria.

II. Time Order

The criterion of time order, because deceptively obvious, is often under-emphasized. All case-control designs, and all cross-sectional designs, collect at once the data both on the supposed cause and the supposed outcome. In such studies, the advent of both cause and outcome is by definition in the past. Their temporal relation cannot be discovered by current observation.

Chronic diseases of insidious onset, in which the timing of initial events is especially obscure, exaggerate the historical problems of these designs. Risk factors or determinants that are personal attributes and change with time—for example marital status, mental disorder, and the relation between them—also obscure time order. So too do predispositions or long latent periods between cause and effect. Conversely, fixed attributes like birthdate or birth order help to fix time order. In postmortem studies of pathology and in ordinary clinical studies, the difficulty is even more marked.

To sum up the contribution to inference of the criterion of time order, if the supposed causal variable can be shown to precede the outcome, then causality is indeterminate but an incentive to exploration; the finding provides grounds for further study of the hypothesis, including analytic elaboration and new independent tests. If the supposed cause and the outcome are observed at the same time and after the event, and if nothing more can be said about time order, the question of causality is likewise indeterminate but has not truly been broached. If the order of the supposed cause and the outcome can be shown to be reversed, however, then one has in hand the most decisive criterion for rejection available. Given falsification by this criterion, the hypothesis at once loses interest and no further criteria need be brought to bear. But in those many instances where the situation is indeterminate, the criterion remains important.

III. Strength of Association

Strength of association refers to the degree to which the supposed cause and outcome coincide in their distribution. It is a statistical cliché that the strength of an association and its statistical significance should not be confused. An association may be weak and yet highly significant. Tests of significance are closely dependent on the numbers in the study, and small differences can be made highly significant by large numbers.

In epidemiology, strength of an association is most commonly stated as a risk ratio, namely relative risk or its surrogate, the odds ratio. The stronger the relative risk for any hypothetical cause, the more likely it is to be causal. This dictum follows from the necessity posed by uncontrolled confounding variables. A confounding variable is one that might give rise to the appearance of an association between the hypothetical cause and the outcome. To achieve this artifact, the variable must correlate with both the hypothetical cause and the outcome under study.

Any confounding variable capable of producing and explaining such an artifact needs to have as strong a relation to the outcome as does the hypothetical cause; when the confounding variable is controlled by design or in analysis, the artifactual association should disappear. Very strong relations are much less common than weak ones in epidemiologic analysis. Thus the stronger the relation, the less a confounding variable capable of explaining the association is likely to exist.

One should perhaps note that the strength of an association is easily suppressed by poor measures of exposure or outcome. While this is properly a matter of research design, epidemiologists must be ready to contend with the situation in which the best available measures—or even the best possible measures—misclassify or give a poor indication either of individual exposure or of outcome. An example in which both exposure and outcome are attenuated is the blurred relationship between life stress as exposure, and mental state as outcome.

To sum up, the stronger an association, the more it supports a causal inference and is affirmative; the weaker an association, the more it is indeterminate. For a given exposure or outcome, incapacity for precise measurement may erode or render indeterminate a true and even strong association.

IV. Specificity

The specificity of an association describes the precision with which the occurrence of one variable, to the exclusion of others, will predict the occurrence of another, again to the exclusion of others. The ideal is a one-to-one relation; in the ideal, a cause is both necessary and sufficient to produce a given outcome. The more closely the relation meets these conditions, the more specific it will be. The more outcomes associated with a given cause, or vice versa, the less singular and specific the relation.

Specificity in the effects of a given causal factor (in the ideal, the cause has only one known effect) can contribute to causal inference in an affirmative way. A causal claim is strengthened especially when a result conforms with a prior hypothesis. For instance, a specific vaccine is expected to protect against a specific disease. In another instance, effects on the risk of miscarriage of environmental factors such as fever were expected and found solely among euploid conceptuses, and not among heteroploid conceptuses nearly all of which are not viable and miscarry spontaneously for that reason.[9]

The absence of specificity, however, in no way negates a causal claim. The fact that penicillin was found to cure a multitude of diseases did nothing to detract from the affirmation of its broad-gauged efficacy. Notwithstanding, many hypotheses—notoriously, the hypothesis that smoking causes lung cancer—have been attacked for the lack of specificity of the effects of the suspect cause. For instance, in adults the meningococcus rarely gives rise to anything but meningitis. That specificity gives the meningococcus no greater claim or plausibility as a causal agent of meningitis than, say, the hemophilus influenza bacillus that also causes meningitis, but which causes a number of other conditions as well.

On the other hand, *specificity in the causes* of a given effect (in the ideal, the effect has only one cause) also improves the plausibility of a causal claim. It is neither a requirement, however, nor definitive when present. That whiteness is specific to swans is a matter of induction; we cannot be sure that a non-white swan will never be found. Likewise, with an effect that seems attributable to only one cause, an additional cause might yet be found. This indeterminacy is a crux of Popper's argument against induction.[4]

But if cola-coloring has been found only in newborn babies of mothers exposed to polychlorinated biphenyl (PCB), that fact does strengthen causal inference, especially when exposure in mothers is confirmed by such other signs as chloracne, and when specificity is enhanced by recurrence in offspring because PCB deposits in the mother's own fat cells may affect subsequent pregnancies.[10] We may say that PCB exposure is sufficient (if not certainly necessary) to the outcome. (This is not to exclude the relevance of the web of factors needed to bring about the exposure; their inclusion or exclusion is strictly a matter of the perspective of the analyst and the frame of reference used.[6])

A cause and effect relation that approaches one-to-one is not infrequently a deliberate scientific creation. As discussed above with the manifestations of phthisis, the artifact follows from the discovery of the effects of some agent and the subsequent reclassification of effects strictly in relation to the agent. In these instances, specificity is the consequence and not the antecedent of the discovery of causes. In other words, with the criterion of specificity, we may be confronted with a problem of time order: did the cause lead to the criterion, or did the criterion itself create the cause?

The evolution of such processes of reclassification offers the clue that specificity can be enhanced. This enhancement points to one of several areas of overlap among the criteria for causal inference—enhanced specificity in turn enhances the strength of association and the strength of the causal claim. This added strength follows from refinements of measurement and definition for both hypothesized cause and outcome; irrelevant "noise" is removed.

Specificity can enhance the plausibility of causal inference even when there is low relative risk.[7] Polio viruses and the meningococcus are the specific causes of paralytic poliomyelitis and meningococcal meningitis respectively. But there are many carriers of these two organisms. Few carriers of polio virus actually contract paralytic poliomyelitis; and similarly, few carriers of the meningococcus actually contract meningitis. Indeed, almost by definition the cases that do occur have not been carriers. This combination of circumstances lowers risk ratios of disease for those exposed to the relevant organism in both these instances. The specificity of the causes of the given outcomes nonetheless renders the associations persuasive, even in the face of low risk ratios.

To sum up, specificity is an affirmative criterion that adds plausibility to a causal claim, but if absent does not detract from it. Specificity in the causes of a given effect is persuasive; specificity in the effects of a given cause usually less so. The criterion overlaps strength of association but is not conterminous with it. Causal and outcome variables well-specified in terms of definition and measurement are essential to achieving both specificity and strength of association, and greater specificity will enhance strength. But specificity of the cause of a given outcome may be persuasive even in the presence of a weak association.

V. Consistency on Replication

The epidemiologist deals with human beings in changing societies; for all practical purposes, variation in the conditions of study is inevitable. The opportunities for exact or nearly exact replication by means of which the physical scientist demonstrates consistency and rules out chance are not available to the epidemiologist.

The epidemiologist's alternative to exact replication is the consistency of a result in a variety of repeated tests. The criterion depends on the persistence of the result in many studies and in many analyses. Consistency is present if the result is not dislodged in the face of diversity in times, places, circumstances, and people, as well as of research design.

A pertinent question is on what grounds consistency is to be decided. To ask for the same risk ratios to recur under many diverse circumstances is to ask for homogeneity, which is certainly to ask too much. Are all studies then equal? The answer to this question requires a qualitative and not a quantitative judgment. A statistical value can be placed, however, on the recurrence of a result in a specified number of replications.

To diminish subjectivity and bias in selecting studies fit to enter a review, objective if qualitative criteria for eligibility need to be set beforehand. Poor execution and analysis must rule out many studies. Aside from discrimination on grounds of design, other sources of inconsistency that must be allowed for reside in the indexes of exposure and of outcome. Irremediable difficulties of measurement are typical of environmental and occupational studies. The access to workers and the work place needed for repeating a study may also prove unattainable. The more public a potential environmental threat has become, the more difficult replication will be.

Consistency on replication is a powerful criterion but one for the long run; it depends on a process. Viewed from a usual perspective, consistency is the epitome of classical induction. Popper's philosophy cannot be reconciled with such a criterion. He would allow that if the hypothesis fails successive tests, it is falsified. But for him every affirmative result in the same direction indicates no more than survival of the hypothesis. These tests merely expand the range of outcomes the hypothesis disallows. They do not affirm or verify, nor alter the probability that a theory is true.

In sum, in the case of a persisting null result, one can agree with Popper that consistency demands rejection of a hypothesis. Indeed, the inductivists Francis Bacon and John Stuart Mill both hold that the elimination of alternatives by negative instances contributes more to inference than does the piling up of positive instances. Yet to "prove" a negative is difficult because alternative qualifying hypotheses are so readily to hand; these render the criterion somewhat less decisive in falsification. In the case of a persisting positive result, I depart from Popper. In my view, consistency is the most powerful verification available.

VI. Predictive Performance

Predictive performance relies on the testing of a deduction. The criterion requires that a hypothesis drawn from an observed association predicts a previously unknown fact or consequence, and must in turn be shown to lead to that consequence.

The characteristics of this criterion—unlisted either by the US Surgeon General's Advisory Committee on the health effects of smoking or by subsequent writers including myself[6,7,11]—add to the difficulty of capturing its contribution to inference about a given association. Although predictive *potential* is inherent in an association, predictive *performance* is not a primary attribute of the initial association itself. Performance follows only from the testing and judging of the hypotheses that can be drawn from the initial association. From the observed association, an *a priori* deduction is made. If the prediction is falsified on testing, the fault may lie, not in the attributes of the observed association, but in the manner of the new test, or in the quality of the inference that led to the prediction. But even if the prediction is borne out, the claim of new knowledge must be cautious. For in either case, several criteria for causation that apply to the initial association will also need to be applied to the predicted association.

The late Imre Lakatos[12] emphasized the importance of this criterion (he called it "excess corroboration") in a philosophical scheme he derived from Popper. (Lakatos' "sophisticated methodological falsification" seems at this point especially to depart far from what he termed the successive developmental phases in Popper of "dogmatic falsification" and "naive methodological falsification." Among Lakatos' many other modifications of Popper, he accepted that successful predictions that yield new facts require verification, whereas Popper accepts only falsification or, more modestly, rejection.) Lakatos took the idea of predictive

performance back as far as Leibniz, whom he cited in these
words:

It is the greatest commendation of an hypothesis (next to
[proven] truth) if by its help predictions can be made even about
phenomena or experiments not tried.[13]

John Stuart Mill, in 1843, recoiled from the predictive idea.

It seems to be thought that an hypothesis . . . is entitled to a
more favourable reception, if besides accounting for all the facts
previously known, it has led to the anticipation and prediction
of others which experience afterward verified.[14]

For Mill, the attempt to establish causality was essentially a
search for proof (in contrast with Popper's search for disproof).
In his view, a consequence that had been anticipated by a theory
carried proof no further than did a consequence that was already
known. John Maynard Keynes added, sharply, that the probability of an outcome predicted by a theory depends on the compatibility of the theory and the given evidence, and cannot be
influenced by when the theory or the evidence was produced.

Against these historic positions, the strength of the criterion of
predictive performance can be seen to derive in part from the
fact that, in accord with Popper's requirement, it is essentially
deductive: by its nature, prediction of new consequences requires an *a priori* hypothesis. *Post hoc* explanations encompass
facts as they exist. As all researchers know, such theories often
fail when tested in new situations. A new situation imposes a
stringent test on a theory; a *post hoc* explanation escapes that
test. For in epidemiology we can be sure that a new situation
will always contain unknowns that a theory may or may not
have accounted for.

While deduction underlies predictive performance, a successful prediction verifies with a force equal to or greater than that
with which a failed prediction falsifies. One example of a successful prediction of new consequences appears in the ever-fer-
tile controversies about smoking and lung cancer. Early critics of
the hypothesis pointed to the apparent immunity of women to

the disease. Defenders countered with observations on the duration of exposure or the latency period before cancer appeared, and on the later adoption of smoking by women than by men. The counter hypothesis therefore predicted that lung cancer rates among later-born cohorts of women would rise. Today we know that women are not immune to lung cancer; in the United States it has equalled and will certainly outstrip breast cancer as the most frequent cancer in women.

Given an *a priori* hypothesis, any research design can be used to test predictive capacity. Among designs, experiments offer the most rigorous tests. Because of the scale and duration of such undertakings, and the ethical issues involved, however, most epidemiologic experiments are designed to verify by confirming existing understanding or associations rather than by predicting new findings. A drug trial will usually be mounted only after the effects of the drug have been observed in laboratories, in animal experiments and in clinical situations. Here by Popper's standards the risk of failure is not high, and a claim of new knowledge might be thought doubtful and not admitted.

On the other hand, a prophylactic field trial may create a new situation. Nutritional supplements may be introduced experimentally where the association of nutritional deficiencies with adverse outcomes provide the baseline datum, as with low birth weight or iodine deficiency disorders. Although the intervention is derived from the previously existing observations, it creates a new situation by repairing a supposed deficiency. Vaccines may be laboratory tested, but when introduced into the community at large, many assumptions must be made, for instance, about the frequency and nature of contacts of infected persons with others and about the spread of organisms in populations. The observed effect in each of these instances constitutes a test of a prediction that can be seen as yielding new knowledge in a new situation created by the experiment.

In summary, predictive performance is a telling criterion. When it clearly produces new knowledge, the *a priori* character of the prediction is strongly affirmative, the more so in that it provides little opportunity for *post hoc* reasoning and avoids many biases that lurk in situations of which the scientist has foreknowledge. Contrary to Popper's falsificationism, in my view a failed prediction often leaves as much room for alternative explanations as a successful one, and therefore may carry no more force in falsifying a causal hypothesis than a success does in affirming one. To determine the success or failure of the prediction, however, all the criteria relevant to judging any association must be applied to the new association.

VII. Coherence

The criterion of coherence is governed by pre-existing theory and knowledge. It requires that an association, to be used as an explanation, coheres with preconceptions about the outcome and about the suspect causal factor. Here too we are dealing with the compatibility of observed results with theoretical deductions, or with inductions from pre-existing knowledge.

We ask ourselves whether the explanation falls into place with the pre-existing structure of knowledge and the hypotheses that follow from that structure. Coherence supports pre-existing theory. Incoherence requires another explanation. If the explanation does not lie in the design or execution of the research, or in some unmeasurable exposure or outcome or in uncontrollable confounding factors, incoherence points to the falsification of pre-existing theory. Incoherence is thereby likely to provoke new theory.

Deduction is involved either way, but only the falsification engendered by incoherence meets Popper's crucial criterion for new knowledge. In contrast, the practicing epidemiologist can usually give no more credence to falsification than to affirmation of theoretical expectations. The coherence of a result with a theoretical deduction is comforting. Incoherence of a result with a deduction is, at the outset, seldom more than discomfitting. By itself an instance of incoherence is often not destructive of an hypothesis. Before a falsifying test leads to the rejection of a theory, matters of design and execution have first to be secured, and support found for the incoherent result in collateral evidence or in replications. Epidemiologic inference rests on a process, and seldom on a single crucial instance.

Pre-existing knowledge poses a test of coherence somewhat different from the requirements of theory. It seems to me that here the testing process must usually involve induction and prove unacceptable to Popper: particular basic facts are used, not as the touchstone within the design of a given experiment or observational study, but as an external criterion in the form of Bacon's induction "by proper rejections and exclusions."

Coherence involves complex judgments, and can be discussed in terms of at least four elements: namely, theoretical fit, factual fit, biologic fit, and statistical fit.

Theory   Findings plausible in terms of pre-existing theory are affirming. When a particular result is implausible—say the fact that cigarette smokers who inhaled seemed to have no greater risk, and sometimes had lesser risk, than those who did not in-hale; or the fact that high protein supplements during pregnancy did not produce anticipated effects on birth weight and instead produced adverse effects—then we have grounds to take pause and to consider rejection of the study result. If, as in both these instances, such a result persists on further exploration, another explanation must be found and theory must be revised or invented.

Facts   When we turn to pre-existing facts, the compatibility of a new result is again affirming. Lack of factual fit has greater weight than either factual fit or theoretical implausibility. Yet it is not always easy to draw a clear line between what is pre-existing fact and what is pre-existing theory, since a test of coherence may require a degree of deduction in both cases. For instance, when a report indicated that in Down syndrome histories of ma-ternal exposure to stressors during pregnancy were of higher frequency than in other pregnancies, the causal explanation of-fered could be decisively rejected from existing knowledge of time order. The theory and facts of organogenesis were sufficient to deduce that the underlying disorder must have arisen before the postulated stresses of a recognized pregnancy.[15] Another re-port took a reduction in the frequency of congenital anomalies at birth as an indicator of improved perinatal health services. This conclusion is incompatible with the known facts, which are sufficient to deduce that virtually all such anomalies arise before most women enter health care for their pregnancies.[16] These examples of incompatible fact exhibit several overlaps among criteria: for example, between theoretical, factual and biological coherence; and between coherence and time order.

Biology The requirement of biologic coherence leaves much room for play in judgments about causality. One man's biologic commonsense is often another man's nonsense.

In normal and abnormal human biology, observations focus on the affected organism rather than on the antecedent factors that might have produced the effect. As a result, their contribution to the understanding of a cause is most often in elucidating the pathways and mechanisms through which a cause may take effect. Besides contributing to coherence, such elucidation can sharpen the specificity, strength and power of a finding, either by specifying conditions under which a process occurs or, mundanely by reducing misclassification of pathologic states that are the outcome. The dengue shock syndrome was clarified once the conditions for its appearance were appreciated, namely, pre-existing immunity to one of three dengue virus types in a pre-pubescent child followed by infection with dengue virus type 2.[17,18]

The search for biologic coherence commonly draws by induction on findings and experiments from species other than human. Such evidence is most useful in constructing theory, but can bear strongly on causal inference. Teratogens provide an example. Teratogens are agents that can produce developmental abnormalities in human offspring, at doses lower than will adversely affect the mother. So far, teratogens found to affect human beings are also teratogenic in at least one animal.[19] It follows that a test of an agent in a large enough range of animals—say seven or more—that proves negative in all species casts doubt on a positive finding in human beings (unless replication should show it to be consistent). Conversely, a positive finding in any one species is verification for a positive finding in human beings.

Familiar problems of animal experiments include the hazards of extrapolation across species and elementary faults in research design.[20] Extrapolation from animal experiments should be cautious for other reasons. Insufficient attention to the design of the animal experiment can result in imprecise transposition to human beings. Winick and Noble[21] inferred from experiments in rats that acute nutritional deprivation early in development resulted in the depletion of brain cells. That result led to many studies in children in deprived environments that attempted to test the effects of early malnutrition on intellectual development. The studies could not and did not in fact test the effects of acute nutritional deprivation; they tested instead the effects of persistent and chronic malnutrition. The results of Winick and Noble were not truly tested in human beings until the effects on development of acute prenatal starvation during famine were studied.[22]

Statistics In science linear relations between causal factors and outcomes are a sort of cultural stereotype for dose-response relations; they signal coherence and verification for virtually all scientists. Any response proportional to dose is strongly persuasive of a causal relation.

It needs to be emphasized that the stereotype is not universal and its absence is not falsifying. Causal relations may take many statistical forms.[6] Some are curvilinear; some may not increase beyond a threshold or may only appear above a threshold; others may be U-shaped parabolas, or S-shaped. It follows that while the presence of a regular dose-response relation is supportive of a hypothesis, its absence has little bearing on whether an association is causal or not.

To sum up, the criterion of coherence with pre-existing theory, fact and expectations is one that always deserves attention. Coherence governs the overall plausibility of findings and ultimately enhances or destroys pre-existing theories. For a given result, coherence usually does no more than afford a modest affirmation of a hypothesis. A strong dose-response relation be-

Figure 1

Criterion		Effect on Hypothesis		
		Supports	Detracts	Indeterminate
Probability Significance				
satisfied	power adequate	+		
	power lacking	+		
unsatisfied	Significance power adequate		+	
	power lacking			+
Time Order				
compatible				+
incompatible			++	
uncertain				+
Strength of Association (relative risk/correlation)				
	very strong	++		
	strong	+		
	weak			+
Specificity in effects of a cause				
	high	+		
	low			+
in causes of an effect				
	high	+		
	low			+
Consistency				
	high positive	++		
	high negative		++	
	low			+
Predictive Performance				
Predicts correctly		++		
Falsifies prediction			+	
Coherence Theoretical				
	plausible	+		
	implausible		+	
Biological				
	coherent	+		
	incoherent		+	
Factual				
	compatible	+		
	incompatible		++	
Statistical				
	dose-response	++		
	other			+

tween causal factor and outcome, however, carries somewhat more affirmative weight than other dimensions of coherence. Incoherence shifts the balance towards rejection. One may also place weight on incoherence as an indicator of falsity where there is clear factual incompatibility between the findings of a study and pre-existing knowledge. Coherence counts most in the overall summing up of a multitude of data.

Conclusion

Conclusiveness in inferring causality—in epidemiology as with all studies in free-living human beings—is a desire more often than an accomplishment. Scientists use both deductive and inductive methods to sustain the momentum of a continuing process of research. Decisive criteria of judgment are available only once in a while. We may follow Popper to the extent of claiming somewhat greater decisiveness for falsification than affirmation, but we cannot do without induction and affirmative tests. The available criteria of judgment, which must nearly always be deployed together, contribute variously to both falsification and verification. The criteria overlap with each other in ways only some of which have been noted. They must be taken jointly as mutually reinforcing; they do not readily form a hierarchy, although some are more forceful than others (Figure 1).

Philosophers of science can and do provide scientists with ideas, stimulation and provocation. When it comes to negotiating the narrows and rapids of research, however, the formalities of philosophy need to be tempered by epidemiologic sense.

References

1. Kuhn TS. *The Structure of Scientific Revolutions.* 2nd ed. Chicago: University of Chicago Press, 1970.

2. MacMahon B, Pugh TF, Ipsen J. *Epidemiological Methods.* Boston: Little Brown Co., 1960.

3. Bacon F. In: Anderson FH, ed. *The New Organon and Related Writings.* New York: Bobbs-Merrill, 1960:99.

4. Buck C. Popper's philosophy for epidemiologists. Int J Epidemiol 1975;4:159–168.

5. Popper KR. *The Logic of Scientific Discovery*. Revised ed. New York: Harper & Row, 1968. Originally published as *Logik der Forschung*. Vienna: Springer, 1934.

6. Susser M. *Causal Thinking in the Health Sciences: Concepts and Strategies in Epidemiology*. New York: Oxford University Press, 1973.

7. Hill AB. The environment and disease: association or causation? Proc Roy Soc Med 1965;58:1217–1219.

8. Jacobsen M. Against Popperized Epidemiology. Int J Epidemiol 1976;5:9–11.

9. Kline J, Stein Z, Susser M, Warburton D. Fever during pregnancy and spontaneous abortion. Am J Epidemiol 1985;121:832–842.

10. Rogan WJ. PCBs and cola-colored babies: Japan, 1968, and Taiwan, 1979. Teratology 1982;26:259–261.

11. Evans AS. Causation and disease: the Henle-Koch postulates revisited. Yale J Biol Med 1976;49:175–195.

12. Lakatos I. Falsification and the methodology of scientific research programmes. In: Lakatos I, Musgrave A, eds. *Criticism and the Growth of Knowledge*. New York: Cambridge University Press, 1970.

13. Leibniz GW. 1678, cited by Lakatos. In: Lakatos I, Musgrave A, eds. *Criticism and the Growth of Knowledge*. New York: Cambridge University Press, 1970:123.

14. Mill JS. 1843, cited by Lakatos. In: Lakatos I, Musgrave A, eds. *Criticism and the Growth of Knowledge*. New York: Cambridge University Press, 1970:123.

15. Stott, DH. Mongolism related to emotional shock in early pregnancy. Vitae Humana 1961;4:57–76.

16. Shapiro S, McCormick M, Starfield BH, Crawley B. Changes in infant morbidity associated with decreases in neonatal mortality. Pediatrics 1983; 72:408–415.

17. Halstead S. The pathogenisis of dengue: molecular epidemiology in infectious disease. Am J Epidemiol 1981;114:632–648.

18. Sangkawibha NS, Rojanasuphot S, Ahandrik S, et al. Risk factors in dengue shock syndrome: a prospective epidemiologic study in Rayong, Thailand. Am J Epidemiol 1984;120:653–669.

19. Brown NA, Fabro S. The value of animal teratogenicity testing for predicting human risk. Clin Obstet Gynecol 1983;26:467–477.

20. Kimmel CA, Holson JF, Hogue CJ, Carlo GL. Reliability of experimental studies for predicting hazards to human development. NCTR Technical Report for Experiment No. 6015. National Center for Toxological Research, Jefferson, Arkansas 72079. January, 1984. Reprinted with permission by the U.S. Department of Health and Human Services, Public Health Service.

21. Winick M, Noble A. A cellular response in rats during malnutrition at various ages. J Nutr 1966;89:300–306.

22. Stein Z, Susser M, Saenger G, Marolla F. *Famine and Human Development: Studies of the Dutch Hunger Winter, 1944/45.* New York: Oxford University Press, 1975.

The Logic of Causal Inference in Medicine

Stephan F. Lanes

Epidemiology Resources Inc.
Chestnut Hill, Massachusetts

It is widely held that scientific knowledge is derived from empirical evidence. Yet not only have scientists failed to find a logical relation between evidence and theory, but some researchers even claim that none exists. Thus, despite the rapid evolution of principles to guide the conduct of medical research, interpretation has remained largely a matter of intuition.

In this paper, I describe the problem of causal inference as it arises in medical science and present a solution first offered by Karl Popper. The perception that we acquire knowledge by accumulating observations until causality becomes established is displaced by the logic of trial and error. In recognizing scientific knowledge as conjecture that can be seen as false, but never as true or probable, Popper explains that uncertainty inherent in all our knowledge and presents a rational way to address it.

1. The Problem of Causal Inference and a Mistaken Solution

Medical scientists are interested in discovering the causes of disease. As Koch said a century ago:

It is not sufficient to establish only the concomitant occurrence of disease and parasite, but the parasite must be shown to be the real cause.[1]

Koch's statement can be framed more broadly by replacing the word "parasite" with a general term meaning any condition considered as a possible cause of disease. In epidemiology, the term "exposure" has developed this connotation.

How can we establish which exposures are causes of disease? This question has been asked in a more general form for many centuries. In 1739, Hume challenged the question's premise:

We are never able, in a single instance, to discover any power or necessary connection, any quality which binds the effect to the cause...we only find that one does, in fact, follow the other.[2]

Hume reasoned that there is no logical way to establish an association as causal because causal associations possess no unique empirical quality. This contention conflicts with the goal of establishing causality that has guided medical science for the past century.[1,3] It also calls into question the scientific basis of the many causes of disease that have been discovered in pursuit of this goal. According to Hume, repeated observation only influences our *belief* that an association is causal. But, since replication carries no implication for validity (because errors may be repeated), our beliefs are without logical justification. The so-called logic of induction, which asserts that through replication we achieve confirmation, is not a logic at all.

The continued search by medical scientists for the empirical qualities that would establish an association as causal[1,4-14] attests to our dissatisfaction with Hume's conclusion that knowledge is merely belief. But none of these efforts has succeeded. The best known of such attempts in modern medicine may be Hill's criteria,[10] the fulfillment of which has been cited by the Surgeon General of the United States as establishing a causal relation between cigarette smoking and lung cancer.[15] After describing many logical flaws in Hill's criteria, Rothman concludes:

These criteria offered by Hill are saddled with reservations and exceptions . . . there are no rules for determining whether an association is causal.[16]

Like Hume, medical scientists have resigned themselves to the conclusion that knowledge must be subjective.[16-18] As one text puts it:

It is not possible to prove causal relationships beyond any doubt. It is only possible to increase one's *conviction* of a cause and effect relationship, by means of empirical evidence, to the point where, for all intents and purposes, cause is established.[19] (emphasis added)

The implications of equating knowledge with belief have gone unappreciated by medical scientists, however, who persevere under the illusion that subjective beliefs can be justified by empirical evidence. Nevertheless, a recent statement about causal inference pertaining to an empirical association between smoking and lung cancer demonstrates that beliefs *per se* are not anchored to empirical evidence:

We're not saying that smoking is not harmful. What we are saying is that there are scientists who *believe* both ways. There is still a debate.[20] (emphasis added)

If knowledge is personal conviction, it bears no logical relation to empirical evidence and can be established only in the mind of the believer. The aforementioned Surgeon General's report[15] exhibits a schizophrenia in its attempt to use Hill's criteria to justify an unjustifiable belief. On the page following the claim that "criteria have been developed to establish causality with a very high degree of scientific probability," the Surgeon General states that "the causal significance of an association is a matter of judgment which goes beyond any statement of statistical probability."

As conceptualized since Hume, knowledge has become divorced from reality. Russell has described the significance of the problem:

It is important to discover whether there is any solution to Hume within a philosophy that is wholly or mainly empirical. If not, there is no intellectual difference between sanity and insanity. The lunatic who *believes* he is a poached egg is to be condemned solely on the ground that he is in the minority.[21] (emphasis added)

The conclusion that knowledge is subjective raises a vital dilemma for medical science. If there is no logical connection between observation and theory, then there is no intellectual reason to conduct scientific research. The belief that smoking causes lung cancer would hold no rational priority over the belief that it prevents lung cancer.

II. *Popper's Solution: A Logical Alternative*

Causality describes but one of an infinite number of possible theories that might explain an empirical association between an exposure and a disease. Thus, data that are consistent with a causal theory do not confirm the theory because the data must also be consistent with competing (noncausal) theories. For instance, the observation that an association between smoking and lung cancer persists after taking the age of study subjects into account does not confirm that smoking causes lung cancer because the association may still be confounded by other (unspecified) causes of lung cancer. Is there no logical conclusion about the etiology of lung cancer that we may draw from this evidence?

We needn't surrender to the notion that knowledge is subjective belief. Popper discloses the escape by posing a deceptively clever question:

Can the claim that a theory is true *or that it is false* be justified by empirical reasons; that is, can the assumption of the truth of observation statements justify the claim that a universal theory is true or that it is false?[22] (emphasis added)

Even though empirical evidence can never show a theory to be true, evidence can show a theory to be false.[23] We cannot justify the statement that smoking causes lung cancer, but we can justify the assertion that certain competing explanations are false. For example, the observation that smoking remains associated with lung cancer after controlling for the effect of age would refute the explanation that the smoking-lung cancer association arises because smokers are older than nonsmokers.

Popper's discovery of the logical relation between observation and theory presents an empirical method of distinguishing which associations are causal. To learn about the causes of disease, we must develop alternative theories to explain associations we have observed. We may then gather observations in an attempt to refute one or more of the competing theories. A scientific theory is a universal statement (i.e., a statement that is abstract in time and place) that makes empirical prohibitions. The empirical implications of a theory serve as tests that may refute the theory. A theory that withstands a potential falsification, because the evidence is found to be consistent with the theory, survives only to be tested again. If we were to generate a true theory, we could never know it with any degree of certainty; a theory can at best be regarded as unfalsified, whether or not it is true.

Thus, we will never realize Koch's ambition to show that an exposure is the "real cause" of disease. Nevertheless, Popper explains the growth of knowledge without relying on confirmation.[24] In our quest for truth, our resources are a boundless supply of explanation and the capacity to uncover misconception. In science, we are interested in finding true explanations, so we should prefer those theories that have not been refuted despite our relentless attempts to do so.[22] The belief that a theory is true will discourage further tests and thereby inhibit the advancement of science.[23] It follows that the goal of medical science should not be to establish causality. As Popper states:

Science never pursues the illusory aim of making its answers final, or even probable. Its advance is, rather, towards an infinite yet attainable aim: that of ever discovering new, deeper, and more general problems, and of subjecting our ever tentative answers to ever renewed and ever more rigorous tests.[23]

III. Solution To a Paradox of Induction

The logical problems of inductive inference by confirmation are well described, if not widely appreciated.[25,26] There is a paradox of induction[27] that can be illustrated as follows. Consider the theory that exposure to a certain virus is a necessary cause of acquired immune deficiency syndrome (AIDS). (By "necessary cause," I mean a condition without which the disease would not occur.) Suppose the details of the theory imply that every AIDS patient harbors the virus. By the rules of induction, to find an AIDS patient harboring the virus is to confirm the theory. The theory also implies that people who do not harbor the virus do not have AIDS. The theory would also be confirmed, therefore, by the observation of a healthy individual who does not harbor the virus. By identical reasoning, however, the observation of a healthy individual who does not harbor the virus would confirm the virus as a necessary cause of every other disease as well. Yet, by studying only healthy people, we would learn nothing about the causes of disease.

The solution to this and other paradoxes of induction is to recognize that knowledge is always theoretical and that evidence that is consistent with a theory does not confirm the theory. Knowledge can advance only by showing that a theory is false. When a theory withstands an empirical test, because an AIDS patient is found to harbor the virus, we may say that the theory has been tested and has not been refuted (Popper used the word "corroborated" to denote that the theory survived a test); but it has not been confirmed.[23] The theory that a certain virus is a necessary cause of AIDS can be refuted only by observing an AIDS patient who does not harbor the virus. Because observations of people who do not develop AIDS cannot refute the theory, such observations are not informative about the validity of the theory.

It is often suggested that although causal theories cannot be proved conclusively, they can be justified as probable. Just as corroboration does not confirm a theory, however, repeated corroboration also does not increase the probability that a theory is true.[23] Consider two theories: the previous example that a certain virus is a necessary cause of AIDS, and a second theory that a particular bacillus is a necessary cause of malignant melanoma. Suppose that we observe a single AIDS patient who harbors the virus. Suppose also that in thousands of melanoma patients, all but the last one are found to have been exposed to the bacillus. If we were to apply probabilistic reasoning to these theories, we would find that the bacillus-melanoma theory, after a vast number of corroborations, would achieve a high degree of probability. It would certainly be considered more probable than the virus-AIDS theory with its lone corroboration. Yet the unexposed melanoma case eventually would show that the bacillus-melanoma theory is false, whereas the virus-AIDS theory may still be true. Probability in this context cannot be construed to have its usual sampling interpretations. We cannot calculate the probability that a theory is true.

IV. A Few Implications

A. Interpretation of Empirical Evidence

Since Hume showed that we can never know that an association is causal, many philosophers and scientists have turned to subjectivism as the only apparent epistemology. Tacit approval of the notion that knowledge is subjective has allowed ambiguous terminology and misguided methods to creep insidiously into the conventions of science. Interpretation is held to be a process that "requires scientific experience and judgment in order to weigh the evidence."[28] When medical scientists consider the evidence of insufficient "weight" to establish belief in a causal theory, causes of disease are referred to as "contributory factors."[15] *A Dictionary of Epidemiology* tells us that a "risk factor" is not a "risk marker" and that neither one is necessarily a "causal factor."[29] It is said that the term "cause" is avoided "because of the lack of certainty in our results."[30]

These contortions of jargon actually reflect uncertainty not about the validity of research results, but about the *meaning* of results (i.e., about interpretation itself). Procedurally, we have relied on the intuitive appeal of confirmation in seeking to establish belief in causal theories by codification and consensus.[18,28,31] Concern with beliefs has permeated a variety of interpretive methodologies. Scientists have developed "causal criteria" in an effort to codify what they believe.[1,4-14] Statisticians of the "frequentist" school offer techniques that attempt to infuse belief directly into the evidence (e.g., procedures for modifying p-values to accommodate the mindset of the investigator before viewing the data).[32] To a Bayesian, probability means "a subjective degree of belief held at a particular time by a particular person."[33] By incorporating belief explicitly into interpretation as the ultimate analytic component, the fashionable Bayesian perspective supposedly "provides for the computation of the probability that a hypothesis is correct."[18] These subjective methods of causal inference survive only on the faith of their followers; they have no empirical foundation.

Causal inference is not a matter of belief; it is a matter of explanation. In science, observations are explained by theories that in turn may be refuted by other observations. Knowledge is not acquired through the depth of one's conviction or the ill-defined "feeling for the data" that is sometimes ascribed to scientists of experience.[31] Knowledge advances by deducing empirical consequences from competing theories and obtaining data that refute one or more of them.

The scientific purpose of gathering empirical evidence is, in principle, to refute one or more of the competing hypotheses that have been put forth as explanations. Interpretation is a matter of distinguishing between the hypotheses that have been refuted and those that remain potentially true. The informativeness of empirical evidence is determined by the hypotheses it refutes. Recognition that knowledge cannot grow through corroborative evidence shifts the focus of interpretation from results ("positive" and "negative" studies) to methods (what alternative explanations were and—especially—were not controlled). This idea has been nicely expressed by Forscher.[34]

The inductivist view that an association becomes established as causal with increasing numbers of replications has familiar counter-examples. There may be no association that has been replicated more frequently than the one between cigarette smoking and lung cancer, yet scientists are still unable to convince those who contend that a causal relation has not been established.[35-38] Conversely, maternal exposure to the synthetic hormone diethylstilbestrol (DES) was accepted by virtually all scientists as a cause of adenocarcinoma of the vagina[39] from the sparse data of a single study.[40]

Instead of asking what aspects of the data can establish causality,[1,4-14] we should ask what other theories could explain the data. All interpretive methods are logically subjugated to this question. The informative aspects of the data are those that show one or more specific explanations to be false. There is a substantial difference in the amount of corroborative evidence between the DES-vaginal cancer association and the cigarette smoking-lung cancer association. The reason that causal interpretations have been offered for both associations is that, thus far, the alternative explanations that have been entertained have all been discarded. This approach to causal inference is fruitfully abetted by unfettered imagination, but it is not susceptible to checklist codification and is independent from beliefs, no matter how prevalent or cherished they may be.

In considering the method of conjecture and refutation, there is one alluring pitfall of which one should beware. Although the logic of falsifiability is straightforward, the practice of falsification is not so clear. One implication is that all knowledge is speculative—including observation.[22]

Indeed, the phenomenon of optical illusions shows that even the most accessible perceptions are filtered through (conscious and subconscious) expectations.[41] Because observations themselves are inferred, it is always possible to deny the truth of otherwise falsifying evidence. In practice, therefore, refutation is never absolute.[23]

It has been suggested that, since refutation is uncertain, the logic of refutability must somehow be faulty.[42-44] This suspicion illustrates confusion between the method and its application.[45] The inevitable uncertainty of all scientific theory is only a problem of methods that seek to establish knowledge. Uncertainty is not a problem shared by the method of conjecture and refutation because conjecture demands no justification. Rather, uncertainty is a logical consequence of this method and is therefore explained by it. The method of conjecture and refutation is how we overcome our uncertainty. For instance, the theory that telekinesis is impossible is empirically refutable, but I suspect there will for some time be considerable doubt about whether it has actually been refuted. The doubt concerns the validity of the relevant empirical observations (as opposed to what they would mean if accepted as valid). This uncertainty can be penetrated objectively by empirically testing alternative explanations for the observations. Whether or not one accepts the observations, the method by which we probe uncertainty is invariant. Unlike induction, which seeks to establish a consensus, the method of conjecture and refutation thrives on criticism.

B. The Limits of Science In Disease Prevention

The method of induction asserts that through an accumulation of data we can establish causation. Under this view, knowledge can attain the status of truth (or its statistical approximation, high probability). Inductivist reasoning suggests that before we utilize a scientific theory, we ought to make sure that it is true. Therefore a crucial question for medical science—one upon which the decision to act is supposed to hinge—is whether the data are sufficient to establish causality:[46-50]

If a causal relation can be considered established, then its implications for practice need to be evaluated.[50]

Thus, acceptance of induction coerces scientists into assuming responsibility for deciding when the evidence is sufficient to provide a basis for action. But causality is never established, so there can be no scientific basis for authorizing policy decisions. Only a belief that a causal theory is true can be established. Therefore, the inductivist principle that guides the application of scientific theories asserts that policy decisions require the subjective approval of scientists. Induction has drawn a mistaken boundary between science and policy.

Consider again the hypothesis that cigarette smoking causes

lung cancer. The claim has been made by scientists that a causal relation between smoking and lung cancer has been established.[15] This statement cannot be justified, however, and has invited skepticism:

> Scientists have developed a theory . . . but it is important to label their belief accurately. It is an opinion. A judgment. But *not* scientific fact. Science is science. Proof is proof. That is why the controversy over smoking and health remains an open one.[51]

By claiming that a causal relation has been established, scientists have initiated an argument they cannot win:

> The tobacco people are quite right: the causal relationship of cigarettes and cancer hasn't been proved; it still is only statistically inferred. The moral is we ought always beware of statistics.[52]

By attempting to justify scientific knowledge with the faith of conviction, scientists have fostered misunderstanding about scientific methods in general and, therefore, about all scientific knowledge.

The misunderstanding can be rectified by presenting scientific knowledge as refuted and unrefuted theory instead of established belief. After purposeful deliberation of the studies on smoking and lung cancer, scientists have offered the explanation that smoking causes lung cancer. The causal theory can be advanced because all of the noncausal explanations that have been entertained have been refuted. Even the barely refutable theory that some unspecified genetic factor causes people to smoke and also to develop lung cancer is undermined by the observations that ex-smokers experience a lower incidence of lung cancer than those who continue to smoke,[53] and by an increased rate of lung cancer among animals randomly assigned to exposure to cigarette smoke.[54] The explanation that smoking causes lung cancer corresponds with the evidence better than all challengers.

Disbelief in the causal theory between smoking and lung cancer is no criticism of medical knowledge, nor will it save smokers from lung cancer. If anyone can offer another explanation for the evidence, then scientists should be eager to test it against the competing causal theory. If no competing alternative can be generated, then, on purely logical grounds, the causal theory is the best available explanation of the evidence, believe it or not.

The scientific evaluation of the validity of a theory should not be confused with the procedure by which we choose to act on a theory. However valid and useful a theory may be, the decision to act on it rests on the *acceptability* of the expected consequences of a variety of possible actions. Policy decisions, therefore, cannot be distilled from science.[55] For example, I know of no untested alternative to the causal theory linking tampon use to toxic shock syndrome (TSS). Even though scientists tentatively accept the causal theory, many women continue to use tampons. The reason—assuming that women are well-informed about the science—is that after assuming the risks of TSS, many women still prefer tampons to the available alternatives. Conversely, the theory that oral intercourse can cause AIDS (by transmitting a virus) is not well tested, but homosexual men have been advised to refrain from the practice for this reason. It is clear that the decision to act on a theory involves a great deal more than the validity of the theory. For one thing, at any time there will usually be many unfalsified theories. Moreover, depending on the objective, even theories that are false may provide a suitable basis for certain actions. Aeronautical engineers, for example, reliably use the theories of Newton even though they have been superseded by those of Einstein.

By asserting that the appropriate time for action is a scientific matter, induction thrusts scientists into the policy arena under a false pretense. Confusion among scientists about the role of science in policy has serious consequences:

The public image of scientists has been distorted by the participation of scientists in public policy formation. . . . When scientists fail to recognize these boundaries, their own ideological beliefs easily becloud scientific debate. If the scientific community will not unfrock the charlatans, the public will not discern the difference—and science and the nation will suffer.[55]

Both science and policy have infinite and constantly attainable goals. Scientists should perpetually search for better explanations, and decision-makers should perpetually weigh the consequences of alternative courses of action. As practitioners, we should receive scientific input, but only to ensure that we appreciate the validity of the theories that guide our actions. As scientists, we should describe the informative studies and furnish the viable theories in an attempt to explain the evidence at hand. Like the theories upon which they are based, decisions can always be reevaluated. Sometimes additional knowledge will cast new light on a previous decision. Discovering that a theory is false (e.g., the theory that thalidomide does not cause birth defects) does not in itself mean that the scientific basis for an earlier decision (e.g., to market thalidomide) was inadequate; all action guided by scientific theory rests on a foundation that may one day be swept away by advancing knowledge.

It has been said that scientists must believe in causal theories to take or propose preventive action.[17] To the contrary, scientists should strive to be agnostic toward their theories, for there is never any reason to believe one's theories are true. The desire to utilize scientific theories should be no deterrent to this position:

It will be argued that society would balk if it knew just how blindly we march into the future. But false reassurances and unjustified confidence will only engender cynicism and destroy credibility.[56]

To ask how much data is sufficient to take action[46-50] reflects misunderstanding about the nature of scientific knowledge and how to use it. Scientists should present explanatory theories, the tests to which they have been subjected and any tests to which they could still be put. Scientists would then invite criticism of theories instead of disbelief. Although we would all like scientific knowledge to be put to good use, scientists have different objectives from practitioners. Science searches steadfastly for the truth, but sometimes untested and even refuted theories are suitable for action. Nevertheless, a theory that survives rigorous tests has attained the highest status of any knowledge; there can be no basis for action that is more secure.[22]

V. Conclusion

Empirical evidence about causal theories in medicine should be interpreted by describing testable, competing explanations. We can distinguish causes from noncauses only by gathering observations that refute one or more of the competing theories. We tentatively infer that an association is causal when a causal theory tenaciously defies our determined efforts to challenge it in empirical competition with noncausal theories. Criteria for "establishing causality" and other methods of subjective inference serve no useful purpose in this process. Faulty observation is always possible, so to invoke unspecified sources of error is unscientific because it does not enable empirical tests. To superimpose subjective judgment, to project a personal conviction beyond the logically testable possibilities, only inhibits further tests that might permit some competing theories to be rationally discarded.

By elucidating the connection between observation and theory, Popper restored scientific knowledge to its empirical foundation. The logic of conjecture and refutation provides a framework for critical exploration that allows us to transform subjective feelings into objective theories. The relation between observation and theory can be communicated, thereby rendering knowledge susceptible to criticism and refutation. In medical science, we may take comfort in recognizing that knowledge is not established. By successfully falsifying our mistaken theories, we may enable people to survive in their stead.

References

1. Koch R. Die aetiologie der Tuberculose. Mitteilungen aus dem Kaiserlichen Gesundheitsamte 1884;2:1.

2. Hume D. *Treatise of Human Nature*. London: John Noon, 1739; revised and reprinted, Selby-Bigge LA, ed. Oxford: Clarendon Press, 1985.

3. Hutchison GB. The epidemiologic method. In: Schottenfeld D, Fraumeni JF, eds. *Cancer Epidemiology and Prevention*. Philadelphia: W.B. Saunders Company, 1982:9.

4. Rivers TM. Viruses and Koch's postulates. J Bacteriol 1937;33:1–12.

5. Huebner RJ. The virologist's dilemma. Ann NY Acad Sci 1957;67:430.

6. Yerushalmy J, Palmer CE. On the methodology of investigations of etiologic factors in chronic diseases. J Chronic Dis 1959;10:27–40.

7. Lilienfeld AM. "On the methodology of investigations of etiologic factors in chronic diseases." Some comments. J Chronic Dis 1959;10:41–46.

8. Sartwell PE. "On the methodology of investigations of etiologic factors on chronic diseases." Further comments. J Chronic Dis 1960;11:61–63.

9. Brollet AJ. On seeking the cause of disease. Clin Res 1964; 12(3):305–310.

10. Hill AB. The environment and disease: association or causation? Proc Roy Soc Med 1965;58(5):295–300.

11. Johnson RT, Gibbs CJ. Koch's postulates and slow viruses of the nervous system. Arch Neurol 1974;30:36–38.

12. Susser M. Judgment and causal inference: criteria in epidemiologic studies. Am J Epidemiol 1977;105:1–15.

13. Evans AS. Causation and disease: a chronological journey. Am J Epidemiol 1978;108:249–258.

14. Weiss NS. Inferring causal relationships: elaboration of the criterion of "dose-response." Am J Epidemiol 1981;113:487–490.

15. U.S. Department of Health and Human Services. The Health Consequences of Smoking: Cancer. Rockville, Maryland: Public Health Service, Publication no. (PHS)82-50179, 1982:16–17.

16. Rothman KJ. Causation and causal inference. In: Schottenfeld D, Fraumeni JF, eds. Cancer Epidemiology and Prevention. Philadelphia: W.B. Saunders Company, 1982:20–21.

17. Susser M. Causal Thinking in the Health Sciences. New York: Oxford University Press, 1973:68–69, 140–141.

18. Miettinen OS. Theoretical Epidemiology. New York: John Wiley and Sons, 1985:330.

19. Fletcher RH, Fletcher SW, Wagner EH. Clinical Epidemiology: The Essentials. Baltimore: Williams and Wilkens, 1982:192.

20. Fishel D. In: Colburn D. Of cigarettes and scientists. Washington Post 1985 May 1 (Health Suppl):7.

21. Russell B. A History of Western Philosophy. New York: Simon and Schuster, 1972:673.

22. Popper KR. Objective Knowledge. Oxford: Clarendon Press, 1972.

23. Popper KR. The Logic of Scientific Discovery. New York: Harper & Row, 1968. Originally published as Logik der Forschung. Vienna: Springer, 1934.

24. Popper KR. Conjectures and Refutations: The Growth of Scientific Knowledge. New York: Harper Torchbooks, 1963.

25. Salmon WC. Confirmation. Sci Am 1973 May:75–83.

26. Gardner M. On the fabric of inductive logic and some probability paradoxes. Sci Am 1976 Mar:119–122.

27. Hempel CG. Studies in the logic of confirmation. In: Foster MH, Martin ML, eds. *Probability, Confirmation and Simplicity*. New York: Odyssey Press, 1966:145–183.

28. Interdisciplinary Panel on Carcinogenicity. Criteria for evidence of chemical carcinogenicity. Science 1984;225:682–687.

29. Last JM, ed. *A Dictionary of Epidemiology*. New York: Oxford University Press, 1983:93.

30. Kleinbaum DG, Kupper LL, Morgenstern H. *Epidemiologic Research*. Belmont, CA: Lifetime Learning Publications, 1982:29.

31. Kolata G. Obesity declared a disease. Science 1985;227:1019.

32. Snedecor GW, Cochran WG. *Statistical Methods*. Ames: The Iowa State University Press, 1980:232–233.

33. Cox DR, Hinkley DV. *Theoretical Statistics*. London: Chapman and Hall, 1974:381.

34. Forscher BK. Chaos in the brickyard [Letter]. Science 1963;142:339.

35. Burch PRJ. The Surgeon General's "Epidemiologic criteria for causality." A critique. J Chronic Dis 1983;36:821–836.

36. Lilienfeld AM. The Surgeon General's "Epidemiologic criteria for causality." A criticism of Burch's critique. J Chronic Dis 1983;36:837–845.

37. Burch PRJ. The Surgeon General's "Epidemiologic criteria for causality." Reply to Lilienfeld [Letter]. J Chronic Dis 1984;37:148–156.

38. Myddelton G. Tobacco and mortality [Letter]. Lancet 1985;1:1430.

39. Stolley PD, Hibberd PL. Drugs. In: Schottenfeld D, Fraumeni JF, eds. *Cancer Epidemiology and Prevention*. Philadelphia: W.B. Saunders, 1982:304.

40. Herbst AL, Ulfelder H, Poskanzer DC. Adenocarcinoma of the vagina: association of maternal stilbestrol therapy with tumor appearance in young females. N Engl J Med 1971;284:878–881.

41. Hoffman DD. The interpretation of visual illusions. Sci Am 1983;249:154–162.

42. Chalmers AF. *What is This Thing Called Science?* St. Lucia: The University of Queensland Press, 1976:60–64.

43. Brown HI. *Perception, Theory and Commitment*. Chicago: The University of Chicago Press, 1977:67–77.

44. O'Hear A. *Karl Popper*. Boston: Routledge and Kegan Paul, 1980:68–80.

45. Popper KR. In: Bartley WW, ed. *Realism and the Aim of Science*. Totowa, NJ: Rowman and Littlefield, 1983:xix–xxxix.

46. Szklo M. The epidemiologic basis for prevention: how much data do we need? Johns Hopkins Med J 1981;149:64–70.

47. Lilienfeld AM, Lilienfeld DE. *Foundations of Epidemiology*. New York: Oxford University Press, 1980:319.

48. MacMahon B, Pugh TF. *Epidemiology: Principles and Methods*. Boston: Little, Brown and Company, 1970:22.

49. Ibrahim MA. *Epidemiology and Health Policy*. Rockville, MD: Aspen Publications, 1985:39–48,101.

50. Mausner JS, Kramer S. *Epidemiology: an Introductory Text*. Philadelphia: W.B. Saunders Company, 1985:191.

51. RJ Reynolds Tobacco Company. Of cigarettes and science [Advertisement]. Newsweek 1985 Mar 3.

52. Kilpatrick JJ. It's still just a row of smoke rings. Boston Globe 1982 Feb 27.

53. Doll R, Hill AB. Lung cancer and other causes of death in relation to smoking. Br Med J 1956;1:1071–1081.

54. Dontenwill WP. Tumorigenic effect of chronic cigarette smoke inhalation on Syrian golden hamsters. In: Karbe E, Parke JF, eds. *Experimental Lung Cancer*. New York: Springer-Verlag, 1974:331–359.

55. Handler P. Public doubts about science. Science 1980;208:1093.

56. Bazelon DL. The judiciary: what role in health improvement? Science 1981;211:792–793.

Scientists and Philosophy

George N. Schlesinger
Department of Philosophy
University of North Carolina
Chapel Hill, North Carolina

Is it important for a scientist to take an interest in the philosophy of science? Not very much if thereby he expects to improve his research technique or problem solving skills. The philosophy of science is of course most intimately involved in science and its methodology, no less than the laws of mechanics that govern the balancing act of the ropewalker have a crucial bearing on the nature of that act. But, just as an acquaintance with the theory of mechanics is virtually useless in facilitating the performance of the high-wire artist, so the study of philosophy is unlikely to contribute much to a scientist's competence.

It is reasonable, however, to suggest that the great importance of philosophy lies in its ability to satisfy an essential need of the contemplative scientist with intellectual curiosity, who seeks understanding for the sake of understanding. In addition to the abstract intellectual gratification, our discipline can also provide an insight into the rational justification, the ultimate significance and metaphysical implications of science, as well as a deeper understanding of the nature of physical reality in general.

Many scientists would refuse to pay much credence to the suggestion that philosophers of science have produced anything that provides deep understanding of the ultimate foundations of science, anything that sheds light on the structure of reality, or indeed anything that may altogether be called a solid discipline. Philosophy, people have complained, lacks any palpable body of knowledge due to the complete absence of any agreed upon, significant conclusions, and in spite of its long history, has accomplished practically nothing, produced no unchallenged results. It seems to belong to an intellectual area where anything goes and perfect anarchy prevails.

It is easy to proffer facts that seem to provide grounds for these misgivings. For instance, in the context of virtually every topic in which philosophers have taken an interest we find some thinker adopting a diametrically opposed position to the one occupied by another, while the majority of their colleagues disagree with both of them. One school of philosophy, for example, has declared particulars—as opposed to the eternal universals—to be transient and insubstantial, while another holds that universals have no real existence at all. To summarize all the intermediate views that have also been championed on this venerable issue would require many pages. It was more than 21 centuries ago, at a time when relevant material was comparatively infinitesimal, that Cicero declared "There is nothing so absurd but some philosopher has said it." One shudders to think what scorching words he would feel impelled to utter if he were alive today.

It is natural to begin our inquiries by asking what might be responsible for this deplorable state of affairs. After all, analytic philosophers make more and more use of rigorous deductive logic in their work, and surely in this domain what is sound and what is not is precisely defined. Thus, with the increase of the application of logical techniques in contemporary philosophical arguments we should have been entitled to expect the imposition of restraints upon the lines of arguments that may be adopted, so that it would no longer be possible to proceed in any fancied direction.

A two-part answer may be suggested. First of all one could say that the controls provided by the rigors of formal logic are insufficient to inhibit the philosopher's flights of fancy, since he is still free to choose wantonly his presuppositions, some of which he may care to articulate while leaving others covertly underlying the initial premises required for his purposes. Being allowed a free hand in the choice of his premises, there is nothing in the rules of logic that is capable of preventing him from reaching any objective that he may be after.

There is a second point, however, the importance of which is somewhat less widely recognized. There are indefinitely many possibilities for committing subtle errors in formal reasoning and it is exceedingly improbable that one could ever safeguard oneself against all the pitfalls that lie along the route leading to the desired conclusion. Of course, formal arguments are widely employed in many disciplines and proneness to error is not a special malady that afflicts mainly philosophers. To err is human, and even a great human being like Einstein was not immune. There is, for example, the famous instance in which the Russian mathematician Alexander Friedmann had pointed out that Einstein's paper on general relativity contained the fatal error of dividing by zero.[1] A radical difference exists, however, between the situation in philosophy and other disciplines. Neither in the physical sciences nor in pure mathematics does the human mind's susceptibility to error have any devastating consequences. In those areas of inquiry virtually any false move that one can make is liable to be detected sooner or later. For example, Einstein arrived through abstract reasoning at the conclusion that the mass of a body increases appreciably when its velocity reaches a substantial fraction of the velocity of light. If his reasoning had been faulty it would have been indicated by the results of the Mössbauer experiment,[2] which illustrated the increase in mass with velocity. Much of mathematics has practical applications and hence invalid arguments can be detected in those cases in ultimately the same way as in the physical sciences. Admittedly, there are areas in mathematics that do not yet have any applications, as is the case with most of number theory. Nevertheless, mathematics offers ready means for the discovery of errors in derivation, the most notable among these being the method of counterexamples. Consider for instance the famous claim made by Fermat that he had discovered a marvelous proof that if *n* is greater than 2, then there are no whole

numbers to satisfy the equation $x^n + y^n = z^n$. No one has succeeded in reconstructing Fermat's proof, and many doubt that
he ever had any such proof. Nevertheless, it is easy to imagine
how one could demonstrate decisively in a line or two that any
alleged proof leading to Fermat's last theorem must be fallacious:
namely, by producing a simple counterexample in which the
equation is seen to be satisfied in a case where $x=a$, $y=b$, $z=c$
and $n>2$.

Philosophers, however, have no resource to such remedies.
No philosophical thesis can be expected to be confirmed or dis-
confirmed by any conceivable experiment. The method of counterexamples is of course widely practiced in philosophical
polemics, but with radically less firm results than in mathematics. It is infected with the infirmities so characteristic to all philosophical discourse. Because of the amorphousness that
permeates the whole discipline, one of the difficulties is that
there is almost always room for disagreement as to whether a
purported counterexample is a genuine instance of the subject
matter under discussion. Suppose, for example, that someone
concluded as a result of an argument he constructed that in general condition C is a sufficient and necessary condition for a person to know that p. Further, suppose that his opponent
produces a counterexample illustrating a situation where I seem
to know that p, even though condition C has not been fulfilled.
In most cases this will not have to be the end of the story, since
the advocate of the original thesis has the option to maintain
that in the situation depicted by his adversary, I cannot in fact
be said to posses a genuine knowledge that p. Decisive results
cannot be produced with the method of counterexamples, simply because the question of what constitutes an instance of
knowledge, or for that matter an instance of freely willed act, or
of a correct value judgment, and so on, is itself disputable.

In mathematics, on the other hand, there is not enough
vagueness to make such countermoves possible. If someone
were to produce a counterexample to Fermat's last theorem that
involved assigning 73 to the value of n, there would be no pros-
pects for fending off his attack by insisting that 73 is not a genu-

ine whole number, or that it is not really larger than 2. The counterexample would settle matters once and for all.

———

Fortunately, the bleak picture that emerges from the foregoing discussion does not accurately reflect the actual situation in philosophy. Admittedly, conflicts among metaphysical theories (conflicts that elsewhere are eventually settled by the accumulation of sufficient evidence) may go on forever. Nevertheless, it does not follow that in philosophy complete chaos is inevitable. Our discipline is not entirely without its defenses against the intrusion of random, arbitrary and capricious arguments, assumptions and theses.

It may be best to cite a few clear-cut, concrete examples to illustrate one of the important ways in which common sense—that has been said to be the knack for seeing things as they are—can provide a mechanism for the rejection of undesirable elements. The examples offer a valid illustration that even in the absence of the resources available in physics and mathematics metaphysics is not altogether bereft of protective means against subtle errors of logic and against the introduction of objectionable assumptions. It depicts the way in which, even before one has been able to put one's finger on it, the presence of an error is brought to our attention through its easily recognizable symptoms.

There is a fairly well known, cunning little argument in favor of absolute fatalism, attributed to some British philosophers who allegedly used it to justify their refusal to take shelter during the bombardment of London by the Luftwaffe. It has sometimes been summarized as follows:

Either I am going to be hurt during this air-raid or I am not. If I am, then all precautions will prove to be ineffective. If I am not, then all precautions will prove superfluous. Thus either all precautions are useless or unnecessary. Hence in any case they are pointless.

It goes without saying that if this argument were valid then it could be used to establish the pointlessness of engaging in any activity whatever purported to promote our welfare. Fortunately, the argument contains a fallacy—the nature of which is of no importance to our present purposes—and hence it is incapable of establishing the fatalistic conclusion. This faulty argument is typical in that regardless how elusive the kind of error of reasoning that has been committed, we find ourselves in a truly fortunate position that virtually guarantees that sooner or later we shall detect the fallacy. In the present case it should at once be obvious why we may feel confident that the argument did go wrong somewhere: the conclusion is radically counterintuitive; practically all the activities we engage in are performed on presuppositions that flatly contradict the doctrine of fatalism. We get out of bed in the morning, supposing that it is both a necessary and useful maneuver that will start us on our way to work, we then go to the kitchen, assuming it to be not a pointless measure for securing breakfast for ourselves, and so on. One is thus alerted to the fact that fatalism is most unlikely to have been correctly established through logically sound steps, by the violent conflict of that doctrine with common sense. And it will be agreed that as soon as we have very strong evidence that a logical fallacy must be lurking somewhere along the (fairly short) process of derivation, then no matter how cunningly it has concealed itself, we are bound to hunt it down through determined effort.

Sometimes when we feel strongly that a conclusion is untenable but have not yet succeeded in locating the error that led to it, we take the existence of such an error for granted and treat the offending conclusion in all our dealings as a false conclusion even though we have never shown it formally to be so. The skepticism throughout history regarding Zeno's famous proof that motion is impossible illustrates this clearly. It has taken some two thousand years before it became feasible to formulate precisely what was wrong with that proof; nevertheless, because of its conclusion's head-on clash with what everyone took to be the incontrovertible testimony of their senses, it was assumed to be fallacious all along. Laymen, scientists and even philosophers kept talking about the swift overtaking the slow-footed and about physical motion in general, as if Zeno never existed.

A considerably less extreme example is provided by philosophers' attitudes during this century toward the doctrine of determinism. Bertrand Russell produced a powerful little argument to show that determinism is a vacuous doctrine.[3] He argued that regardless what our universe is actually like, it is quite a trivial task to construct functions that will describe the behavior of all the physical systems we have observed. All we need to do is compile a list of the corresponding values of any two variables at various points in time and this list will automatically furnish a mathematical function satisfied by all our data. Of course, the more data we shall have recorded the more complex the function is likely to be, and after some stage the complexity will be so immense that the resulting expression may cease to be of any practical use, but that is insufficient reason to disqualify it from being an actual law of nature. And just as we would regard a weather bulletin that said "Tomorrow it will either rain or it will not rain" to be utterly vacuous because there exist no circumstances under which it could turn out to be false, so the assertion that the universe is strictly deterministic, which is inevitably true no matter what, can be of not the slightest interest to us.

Russell's argument has not proven easy to refute and indeed until this very day no generally accepted answer to it exists. Remarkably enough, in spite of it, between the time he first advanced his thesis at the beginning of this century and today many hundreds of papers have been written discussing the issue of determinism and its important implications; millions of words have been used to show that contemporary physics implies (or does not imply) an indeterministic universe, or to show how free will can or cannot be reconciled with strict determinism. But surely if Russell is right, all these discussions are absolutely pointless!

How do we account for the strange fact that many philosophers have gone on with their arguments concerning determinism and its ramifications after Russell precisely as before? The answer is, of course, what we said earlier: there exist beliefs so deeply entrenched that when a seemingly conclusive argument produces a strongly counterintuitive result implying their falsity, it is at once assumed that the argument is bound to be wrong and eventually it will be proven to be so. The belief that there is a radical difference between a universe where everything is an inevitable consequence of what went on before, where the laws of nature dictate exactly what will and what will not take place, and a universe that permits spontaneity, where a genuine chance event may materialize anywhere at any time, is one such belief deeply rooted in our minds. Therefore it has been taken for granted that sooner or later an adequate way to reply to Russell will be found that will vindicate our strong intuition that the issue of determinism is of great significance.

———

Thus Cicero may have been right about philosophers who have indeed from time to time attempted to foist upon us some outlandish ideas. Cicero's criticism, however, does not imply the complete breakdown of philosophy as a discipline, where anything goes and complete lawlessness prevails. There are several reasons why philosophers may come forward with fancy-bred suggestions. First of all, a bizarre thesis may have a shock value. Through its dramatic power it may succeed in counteracting the effects of some entrenched thesis that has erred in the opposite direction; it may serve as a source of illumination, since through exaggeration it may magnify the finer features of the truth that might otherwise be too subtle and escape notice; it may suggest new directions and lines of approach; or, it may simply act as an irritant and goad others into reacting to it sharply and thus generate a lively debate in the course of which useful ideas may surface, and so on.

Weird theses and arguments are, as we know, occasionally advanced on the assumption that asserting the precise opposite of what everyone regards as the plain truth, amounts to originality. Then again, as David Stove has pointed out[4] in his delightfully witty, devastating criticism of whom he calls the "four contemporary irrationalists" (Popper, Lakatos, Kuhn and Feyerabend), with the inauguration of the Jazz Age some philosophers have adopted Cole Porter's lyrics "day's night today . . . good's bad today" as their regular policy, anticipating that by standing ideas on their head they will succeed in lending matters an exciting enough appearance so as to attract attention to our unduly neglected discipline. Indeed, regardless of what one may think of the achievements of these authors, one will have to concede that they did succeed to give their ideas wide circulation among scientists.

Ultimately, however, theses that represent gross distortions of the truth are not likely to remain a part of our system of beliefs. They often remain so for a while because it takes some time before all the ramifications of a new idea are revealed and its significance becomes evident, or simply because an untenable idea is buttressed by such ingenious arguments that it becomes difficult to recognize its precise nature. Nevertheless, when a thesis deviates to a marked degree from what sober and reasonable people sense to be a plausible description of the way things are, that will as a rule make its transience highly probable.

During the last few years philosophy of science has certainly received its fair share of attention grabbing, tantalizing, novel theses. We have been told that in science old theories are overthrown and replaced not because of any objective reasons, but as a result of social pressure or because of some subjective and arbitrary reason; that scientists are not in the business of discovering the truth, they are merely trying to get hold of whatever may be available as means for the manipulation of nature; that what we observe is not determined by external reality but by the theories we happen to subscribe to since our theories are the spectacles that determine what we see—without them we see nothing definite; that as taught by extreme nominalists, much of what is naively taken to be part of objective reality is actually dependent on what language we happen to be speaking. Thus while to us it may seem beyond doubt that no green surface is identical in color to any blue surface, those who speak a language in which anything colored green before time t, or colored blue after t is called "grue," are fully entitled to think otherwise.[5]

For a while such ideas may be found refreshing and even daringly innovative. Sooner or later, however, their appeal wears off and they are recognized for what they are.

Thus, Cicero may have been right in what he said about philosophers. For one reason or another they have indeed suggested a great deal of absurdities. The good news, however, is that the value of philosophy on the whole has not as a consequence been jeopardized. As we have already indicated, radical opinions, even when untrue, may have merit in that they are capable of serving as effective antidotes to some strongly held prejudices. More importantly, most of such opinions are unlikely to gain permanent foothold in our system of beliefs. Theses that flagrantly misrepresent reality are likely to be discredited because they, or at least their ramifications, will offend our sensibilities too strongly.

Thus it is in good conscience that one may recommend to the empirical scientist to stand back occasionally and engage in philosophical reflection upon the ultimate nature and significance of his enterprise. He should find it worthwhile to study philosophical literature, for it contains matters of substance that may provide insight and intellectual satisfaction.

Nevertheless, it is vital to realize that there are additional factors to consider. While it would be a mistake to expect from one's philosophical studies direct practical help in one's struggle with day to day problems, such studies can provide a more balanced perspective, a guidance for general orientation and a means for thought organization that may translate into practical benefits as well. To illustrate this point I shall confine myself to a short discussion of a single example, but one that involves a topic of genuine significance, the topic of the intelligibility of nature.

Recall Einstein's famous saying that the most incomprehensible thing about nature is its comprehensibility.[6] Indeed, an enormous amount of mental effort has been required for the great accomplishments of the leading physicists throughout the ages; nevertheless, many of them found their work almost unbelievably easy compared with what they thought one had a right to expect. After all, nature is infinitely rich; time and space seem endless, teeming with myriad events, processes, particles and complex physical systems exemplifying an immense variety of properties, and yet we have succeeded in understanding so much about these in relatively such a short time. It is as if nature has gone out of its way to help us to unravel its secrets.

It is mostly great scientists like Galileo, Kepler, Newton and Einstein, and not professional philosophers who have commented and marvelled about the surprising intelligibility of nature. In the prevailing intellectual climate many philosophers wish to have little to do with notions of a "helpful nature" and the like, with which they feel very uncomfortable. To offer one concrete illustration of a crucial aspect of reality that has made the scientist's task immeasurably easier than it otherwise would have been, let me allude to the astounding relation that exists between abstract mathematical discoveries motivated by no practical purpose and the empirical laws of nature. One of the most dramatic examples involves the striking application of the curves known as the conics. There are four different sort of curves in which a plane cuts a cone. One is the circle, when the cross-section is perpendicular to the axis of the cone; another is the ellipse, when the cross-section is somewhat tilted. When the cross-section is further tilted so that it becomes parallel to one of the lines of the surface of the cone, the parabola is generated. Finally, those planes that cut both the upper and the lower halves of the cone produce a curve in two pieces, the hyperbola.

The Greek geometricians beginning with Appolonius of Perga became fascinated by this family of curves and succeeded in working out many of their important characteristics. Their interest was purely intellectual and aesthetic; there was no intention to apply the results to any practical problem. Eighteen hundred years later, however, Kepler discovered that the orbits of planets are of an elliptical shape. Not much later, it was found that the trajectories of heavy objects near the surface of the earth describe a parabola. Finally it was discovered that comets follow a hyperbolic path. Of course, there are infinitely many kinds of curves. We are thus unbelievably fortunate that three of the most important kinds of movement happen to take place along the infinitesimally small fraction of curves that ancient geometricians have already subjected to meticulous study, thus placing us in the advantageous position of being thoroughly acquainted with them.

Some time ago the mathematician, physicist and Nobel laure-

ate Eugene Wigner delivered a lecture entitled "The Unreasonable Effectiveness of Mathematics in the Natural Sciences" in
which he said:

> The miracle of the appropriateness of the language of mathemat-
> ics for the formulation of the laws of physics is a wonderful gift
> which we neither understand nor deserve.[7]

Thus we see a great scientist filled with a sense of gratitude
for the fact that in spite of there being infinitely many possible
universes, the actual universe happens to have such an exceedingly rare and singularly precious future. There are many, however, who are wary of mysteries and will definitely not tolerate
miracles, and who have gone out their way to show that none
exists. For example, in his very enjoyable book, M. Guillen
claims that "the mathematical imagination is a sixth sense" that
enables us to learn about our surroundings and thus cope with
it. He says:

> . . . it seems . . . that the mathematical imagination is an extra
> sense with which we can perceive the natural world. And it is
> an extremely efficacious sense, because it often perceives reality
> long before our scientific senses do. If thought of it this way, the
> coincidence between the natural world and the mathematical
> world is not any more mysterious than the coincidences between
> the natural world and the auditory, tactile and olfactory senses.[7]

That a highly intelligent person should resort to such an illu-
sive argument vividly illustrates how unwelcome anything that
smacks of the notion of a "solicitous" nature is to some minds.
Surely the analogy with the highly useful five senses that we
have been blessed with is entirely misplaced. The striking usefulness of mathematics would be just as puzzlesome if human
beings never existed. After all it has nothing to do with the fit-
tedness of our faculties that tensor calculus happens to be applicable to general relativity or Hamilton space to quantum
mechanics. Also, of course, those important kinds of trajectories
that exemplify the conspicuously unique feature of having the
shape of curves generated by the intersection of a plane and a

right round cone had this feature before the emergence of any species capable of becoming aware of the fact.

Gullien's response, however, is a typical instance of the widespread reaction to the centuries-old belief that the sole concern of the entire universe is man, the crown of creation; that nature is an instrument of a willed force and every event is a result of a cosmic desire to please or tease us. The currently dominant attitude represents a continuing backlash fueled by a fierce determination to reject any idea that smacks of the suggestion that the universe may be having any animistic or teleologic elements.

Against this it should be stressed that there is virtually limitless scope to investigate those features of the universe that have unquestionably facilitated the progress of science without ascribing any plan or purpose behind nature's laws and without in the least implying that any of our findings require or make it appropriate for us to have sentiments of gratitude or admiration. Let me illustrate this idea using another group of remarkable features shared by many of the laws of nature that we have succeeded in formulating.

It has been often pointed out that the most basic laws of nature, like Newton's laws of gravity, are exceedingly simple and thereby lend themselves to easy discovery. There are, however, far less obvious factors that have been crucial to the unravelling of nature's secrets. For example, we may regard ourselves as singularly lucky that the configuration of planets happens to be such that the relatively simple law of attraction governing two bodies is not masked to any appreciable degree by the interference of a third body. This arrangement permitted Newton to make the immensely simplifying assumption that the motion of each of the planets was shaped by only one other attracting body. The formidable problem of many-body-attraction could thus await the mathematical work done in the second stage of development. Had it been necessary for Newton to deal with it right from the beginning, the complex planetary orbits would have been unlikely even to offer him a clue that this problem had a relevance to his task.

Just as fortunate is the fact that the deviation of actual gases from the behavior of ideal gases at normal temperatures is of a small enough order to permit first the discovery of Boyle's law, without which the much more complex Van der Waal's law might never have occurred to anyone.

This particular aspect of nature, namely, the separability of its various features that renders its secrets discoverable serially, seems to be a more significant factor in making the world intelligible to us than the simplicity of its basic laws. After all in the absence of the latter, nature might have still yielded its secrets to a greater effort and intelligence; however, if the different aspects of natural phenomena too much interfered with one another, then regardless how simple each law on its own might have been, these could have so completely masked each other as to prevent altogether their discovery by rational means.

Most people would readily grant that there is probably scope for discovering innumerably many laws of nature that could be shown to have remained forever inaccessible to us were it not for the fact that various phenomena were sufficiently kept apart so that their interference with one another could at first be ignored. It is also fairly obvious that such an investigation can be carried on without believing that it is justified or even merely meaningful to ascribe any purpose or reason to explain why nature has been arranged the way we find it. Furthermore, regardless how impressive the results, it still does not follow that nature on the whole is intelligible. It may well be that the entire body of contemporary scientific knowledge is but an infinitesimally small fraction of what there is to know. All we can say is that compared just with what was known as recently as 300 years ago, an immense variety of phenomena have become intelligible to us.

I may thus conclude with a somewhat fuller statement of the reasons why scientists in general and the epidemiologist in particular should want to take an interest in philosophy. First of all there is a chance of partaking at least to some degree in the experience of mental exhilaration of which it has been said that no one on whom nature or study have conferred the capacity to delight would purchase the gifts of fortune by its loss. To the scientist *qua* scientist, however, more specific considerations exist as well, an instance of which is illustrated by this section's discussion. A thorough investigation of the various aspects of reality that have facilitated our rapid understanding of nature's laws may have a profound impact on the scientist's practical conduct. This impact would especially affect those who work in the health sciences where, unlike physics, very few laws have so far been discovered that are as fundamental, simple, universally applicable and able to unify vastly diverse phenomena as, for example, the laws of Newton or Maxwell. Realizing that though nature is subtle she is not mischieveous, and there are no forces out to frustrate our efforts, we should feel inspired to continue our search for laws that have so far eluded us. The belief that we are living in a "user friendly" universe should sustain us in our scientific endeavours, confident that they will yield vast results in comparatively short time.

References

1. *Isaac Asimov's Book of Facts*. New York: Bell, 1981:146.

2. Kerwin L. *Atomic Physics*. New York: Holt, Rinehart, & Winston, 1963:111.

3. Russell B. *Mysticism and Logic*. London: Pelican, 1963:146.

4. Stove, D. Karl Popper and the Jazz Age. Encounter 1985 June:65–74.

5. Schlesinger GN. *The Intelligibility of Nature*. New Jersey: Humanities, 1985:Appendix A.

6. Schlesinger GN. *The Intelligibility of Nature*. New Jersey: Humanities, 1985:xiii.

7. Guillen M. *Bridges to Infinity*. Los Angeles: JP Tarcher, 1983:71.

COMMENT

Probability Versus Popper: An Elaboration of the Insufficiency of Current Popperian Approaches for Epidemiologic Analysis

Sander Greenland

Division of Epidemiology
UCLA School of Public Health
Los Angeles, California

In his contribution to this volume, Weed[1] has put forth a "Popperian" evaluation of Hill's criteria for assessing causal inference. Elsewhere, he has eloquently described and prescribed a Popperian approach for the general problem of causal inference in epidemiology.[2] In both contributions, he criticizes the notion that either causal inference or rational decision making should be approached with methods founded on concepts of judgment, belief, opinion, or subjective probability. (Lanes, in this volume, expresses similar sentiments, although his presentation suffers from inaccurate representations of other viewpoints, as described below.) I will here argue for the hypothesis that the conflict between Popperian and more judgment-oriented epidemiologists such as Susser[3,4] arises from the failure of both sides to distinguish the needs of the branch of science called epidemiology from the needs of the branch of public health called epidemiology. I will further argue that the Popperian methods[1,2,5] proposed thus far fail to meet all the needs of either decision making or inference, and so as yet require epidemiologists to fall back on other methods. In other words, though Popperian methods may be necessary for good scientific or decision analysis, none of the Popperian approaches described so far constitutes a sufficient system for such analyses. This point was, I believe, conceded by Maclure,[5] but not elaborated by any of the Popperian epidemiologists.

The Needs of Public Health

Epidemiology as a science is not inherently concerned with anyone's opinion about how things are, but only how things are. It is thus understandable that Popperian epidemiologists wish to identify as scientific only statements about nature (and then only certain types), and reject from science individual beliefs or opinions about such statements. It is equally understandable that a sound methodology for practicing the science of epidemiology will be found inadequate for practicing the public-health profession of epidemiology: public health is not a science, but a form of social activism, one whose benefits appear profound enough to society that it is institutionalized and heavily subsidized by governments. A public-health activist promoting or searching for an action will be concerned with communicating his or her own opinions, evaluating the opinions of colleagues, and influencing the opinions of governmental figures and the public.

Weed[2] glances in this direction with a citation from Alexander Bain: "Belief has no meaning except in reference to our actions." To understand the needs of the activist, consider the partial converse that action must be evaluated with reference to (among other things) our beliefs. For example, why has there been such a drive from the public-health profession to somehow curtail the promotion and consumption of cigarettes? Only a fairly strong belief that cigarette use frequently causes illness and death can motivate such a pursuit. And only the transmission of that belief to governmental figures can lead to governmental actions, such as mandatory labelling.

If one accepts the thesis that belief is a critical element in motivating and carrying through actions, the classical criteria for causal inference may be evaluated in terms of how well they serve to orient beliefs toward the best available scientific explanation of the observations at issue (I suspect that for "best available" a Popperian would substitute "most corroborated"). In this regard, Weed's[1] analysis of Hill's criteria remains relevant even if we remove those criteria from the realm of scientific inference to the realm of decision making, for his analysis clarifies the utility of the criteria in finding the best available explanation. But motivation for action, either in emotional or risk-benefit terms, remains absent. Could the activist successfully motivate his own or anyone else's action by adopting a purely critical attitude, as Weed recommends?[1] I think not. Imagine a cigarette warning label that read: "The hypothesis that cigarette smoking is hazardous to health is at present the best available explanation for observations to date, but like all such theories it should not be regarded as established."

The role of judgment and belief in motivating action is amply attested to in the public-health literature. Consider the controversies presented by Susser.[4] Each of these conflicts of opinion pivoted around an impending public-health decision: whether to employ mass vaccinations (typhoid, polio), or whether to attempt to influence individual behavior (cigarette smoking). (The extensive literature on causal criteria cited by Weed[1] was largely inspired by the cigarette-lung cancer controversy, in which an action had to face resistance from a powerful industry and strong individual addictions.) Popperians may "morally" object to the entry of irrational elements into these conflicts, but attempts to banish such elements from the environment in which public-health decisions are made are at best naive.

The Purpose and Utility of Subjective Bayesian Analysis

Decision Making   Leaving aside irrational elements of motivation, and focusing instead on rational decision making, critical rationalism (and science in general) provides no advice as to what degree of "corroboration" is an action level (indeed, Popperian epidemiologists provide no numerical scale for corroboration). Likewise, a purely critical approach to decision making provides no clue as to how one should weigh risks and benefits against one another in making a decision. Yet, the risks and benefits of an action must be weighed, with the action dictated when benefits outweigh risks and costs. Given the uncertainty about the consequences of most actions, I believe it inevitable that concepts such as "expected utility" will enter into decision making, and with them the notion of subjective probability. Although Weed[1] points out some shortcomings of using *only* subjective probability in decision making, he offers no compelling reason not to employ it there, and the method will remain useful to persons who need a method of rationally allowing new data to influence their beliefs and actions. In fact, a whole field of Bayesian decision analysis has grown up in response to the latter need[6]—although the primary area of application has been in business administration, not public health. This theory does provide an explicit means of weighing risks and benefits. And as long as those who oppose the use of probability in decision making fail to provide an alternative means of explicitly weighing risks and benefits, probability will remain a fundamental component of decision analysis.

Scientific Inference It is in Popperian discussions of scientific inference that subjective probabilities are most strongly rejected.[2] Subjective probabilities are statements about an individual's beliefs (as opposed to statements about theories, or theories about beliefs), and so by Popperian standards are not scientific statements at all. I believe Popperians should require no more justification than this for banishing subjective probability from science; nevertheless, some press their attack with accusations of internal inconsistency against all subjective probability systems.[2] Such accusations stem not from some inherent logical inconsistency in the concept of subjective probability, but from an improper identification by some Popperians of all subjective probability theories as subjective theories of truth or theories of induction (an error *not* committed by Popper[7]), and a failure by some discussants (including some promoters of subjective and inductive systems[8]) to adequately distinguish statements about theories from statements about individual beliefs when making deductive arguments regarding scientific hypotheses. For example, in Miettinen's comment[8] that Bayesian analysis "provides for the computation of the probability that a hypothesis is correct," "probability" refers to *one's belief* about the correctness of a hypothesis, not, as Lanes[9] misinterprets it, to some "ultimate analytic component" of causal inference, or to *the correctness of the hypothesis itself.* (Such misinterpretation is no doubt encouraged by the use of phrases like "the probability" rather than *"one's* probability.") Popperians like Lanes fail to grasp the logical foundation of Bayesian methods because they fail to grasp the Bayesian distinction between an individual's probability of a hypothesis (which is a statement about belief, varying from individual to individual) and the truth value of a hypothesis (which is either true or false, independent of anyone's belief). Their confusion is enhanced by the fact that a Bayesian analysis hypothetically entertains different possible states of nature, since nature is (presumably) capable of influencing beliefs, e.g., through data. Nevertheless, Bayesians are as aware as Popperians that one's beliefs about a scientific theory do not affect the correctness of that theory.

To illustrate the lack of parallelism in reasoning about theories and beliefs, suppose A is a scientific theory, B is a prediction about the observable world (e.g., the outcome of an intervention program), and consider the valid deductive form, *modus ponens*:

Premise: A implies B
Premise: A is true
Conclusion: B will be true

Now consider the deceptively parallel argument:

Premise: Karl believes that A implies B
Premise: Karl believes A is true
Conclusion: Karl believes B will be true

This is *not* a valid deduction: to deduce the conclusion we must assume (in addition to the stated premises) that Karl thinks in a logically coherent manner, and that Karl has bothered to put together his beliefs (the premises) and make the deduction. At most, the argument is a lesson for Karl about what he ought to believe about B, given his other beliefs: one may argue that Karl, as a true scientist, ought not to believe that A is true, but *if* Karl does commit this sin and also believes A implies B, we would consider his thinking irrational if he also believed B will not be true.

Analyses (such as just given) of what constitutes rational belief systems are what Bayesian subjective probability theory is about; in particular, it is about how one assigns probabilities (meaning: degrees of belief) to hypotheses in a logically coherent manner, *given* that one is making such probability assignments at all. For example, Bayesian theory finds that *if* Karl considers two mutually exclusive hypotheses G and H, and assigns to them probabilities $P(G)$ and $P(H)$, *then* the only rational or coherent value that Karl can assign to the probability of the hypothesis "G or H" is $P(G) + P(H)$ (just as Karl's only rational belief for the status of B, given his other beliefs, was "true"). In fact, it can be shown that to be coherent, subjective probability assignments must follow all the rules of mathematical probability.[10] Note that, in this analysis, no reference is made to the objective truth of G or H, nor is any hypothesis deduced or "induced" from the data.

Rational analysis of beliefs has an important use in epidemiologic science, especially in the form of subjective Bayesian analysis. I do not believe such analyses can or should substitute for Popperian methods, but they can be applied as a parallel activity. Robins and I have described their utility elsewhere:[11] basically, they can serve to scrutinize the assumptions underlying typical statistical analyses.

Scientists (including Popperians) often analyze their data ignorant of strong and unjustified assumptions underlying their analytic methods. Bayesian analysis can make clear the assumptions hidden in one's analytic methods, and allow one to see the strength of one's data relative to commonly used analytic assumptions.[11] This clarity comes from expressing analytic assumptions (such as assumptions about confounding, effect modification, and dose response) as prior distributions, and seeing how sensitive posterior distributions are to shifts in those priors. With such sensitivity analyses, one may discover that one's data are weak relative to common analytic assumptions, and thus get a better sense of the caution required in employing any assumptions or models in one's data analysis. Sensitivity analyses may of course be constructed out of frequentist computations; in fact most authors (including Robins and me) resort to such computations. But the Bayesian perspective allows one to make sense out of (or reveal as nonsense) many computations that are all too often performed blindly.[11]

Popper devoted some space in *The Logic of Scientific Discovery*[12] to criticizing the type of Bayesianism prevalent in the early 1930's, when the book was written. This form of Bayesianism, originally promoted by Keynes and (later) Jeffreys, and now known as "logical" or "necessarist" theory, does indeed have an inductivist element quite antithetical to Popper's main thesis. It has, however, been largely supplanted by the type of subjective Bayesian theory found in de Finetti[10] and Savage,[13] which treats probabilities as individual psychological constructs used to guide one's own betting behavior or predictions. In this theory the probabilities involved are "rational degrees of belief" only in the sense of consistency of assignment, as described above; they are not necessarily rational with respect to all available knowledge, and so should not be confused with the "rational degrees of belief" of necessarist theory. Both Popper *and* modern subjective Bayesians regard the necessarist theory (and inductive probability) as unacceptable, insofar as it appears to produce "knowledge out of ignorance."[7] Popper is also critical of the modern subjective Bayesian view, but the main force of his argument seems to be empirical: he holds that such theory cannot account for (and has no logical connection to) the success of the physical interpretation of probability in physics.[14] The controversy is too involved to cover here; suffice it to say that the issue is far from resolved.[15]

The Challenge to Popperian Epidemiologists

Popperian writers in epidemiology have thus far been amazingly uncritical in their continued use of conventional statistical methods. Having failed to draw any sound logical connection between Popperian methods and the frequentist rituals they (like everyone else) perform on data, they also fail to point out that use of frequentist statistics automatically enters "chance" into the roster of possible explanations for conflict of observations with predictions. Weed[1] even states that "probability may be reasonably incorporated into our ontological battery (e.g., as the random alternative to causality)." Yet, by the criteria given by Weed,[2] chance is a decidedly poor and even unscientific explanation of anything: it does not lead to more precise predictions; it does not explain previous observations in more detail; it does not suggest new tests; it certainly does not provide a unified explanation of phenomena previously thought unrelated; and it is not even ultimately refutable (no matter how small the p-value is, it is always possible the deviation was "due to chance"—and in typical epidemiologic situations, the p-value will rarely be essentially zero). In essence, the "chance" explanation is a means of invoking unspecified sources of error to protect the tested hypothesis—a process that Lanes[9] calls unscientific.

Popperians should give credit to subjective Bayesians for treating the "chance" explanation for what it really is: a covert (and perhaps irresponsible) way of admitting that conflict between particular observations and predictions of essentially correct theories may occur as the result of our inability to take account of all conditions that determine what we observe. I call this inability *the* statistical problem. To a subjective Bayesian, labelling a result as due to "chance" or "random" variation is analogous to diagnosing an illness as "idiopathic," in that it is just a way of making ignorance sound like technical explanation.

The inadequacy of frequentist statistics in dealing with unaccounted-for determinants of observations is amply illustrated in nonrandomized epidemiologic studies. It is not difficult to find studies in which the crude confidence limits entirely exclude the estimate obtained after control of one or two key confounders, and in which only the crude result corroborates the causal hypothesis at issue.[16] Had the key confounders *not* been measured in those studies, the crude confidence limits would have been entirely misleading as to the confounding produced by the unaccounted-for determinants. A Bayesian analyst could do better by employing a prior distribution that included parameters for the associations of the unmeasured confounders with the study variables (of course, if the very existence of the confounders was unsuspected this alternative would not be available).

If one rejects any and all uses of subjective methods (such as subjective Bayesianism) in causal inference, it becomes one's responsibility to lay out an alternative solution to the statistical problem, rather than continuing (like everyone else) to fall back on vague or inaccurate interpretations of p-values and confidence intervals. In particular, Popperians need to develop their own general criteria for determining when a particular observation contradicts or corroborates a given epidemiologic theory, and when a particular epidemiologic study design is capable of discriminating between competing theories. Weed[2] and Maclure[5] have made a start in this direction, but the task I am talking about is far more extensive; among other things, it requires justifying the means by which one assesses precision and uncertainty. In other words, those who reject subjective methods must elaborate a new and coherent theory for study design and analysis, one that is logically consistent with and explicitly serves what they see as the proper role of scientific research in causal inference. Although some elements of this theory may resemble earlier approaches, such a theory should not be a mere patchwork of tools borrowed from predecessors (such as Neyman-Pearson theory). And to be true to their own philosophy, the developers should derive and present refutable predictions from the theory.

In closing, I would like to reiterate that I do not question that Popper's philosophy contains much of value for causal inference; but I also believe that it is grossly insufficient to prevent us from being "more wrong than we need be."

Acknowledgments

I would like to thank Charles Poole for his criticisms of this paper, and Evalon Witt for word processing.

References

1. Weed DL. Causal criteria and Popperian refutation. In this volume.

2. Weed DL. On the logic of causal inference. Am J Epidemiol 1986;123:965–979.

3. Susser M. Falsification, verification, and causal inference in the light of Sir Karl Popper's philosophy. In this volume.

4. Susser M. Judgement and causal inference criteria in epidemiologic studies. Am J Epidemiol 1977;105:1–15.

5. Maclure M. Popperian refutation in epidemiology. Am J Epidemiol 1985;121:343–350.

6. Lindley DV. Making Decisions. 2nd ed. New York: Wiley, 1985.

7. Popper KR. Probability magic or knowledge out of ignorance. Dialectica 1957;11:354–374.

8. Miettinen OS. Theoretical Epidemiology. New York: Wiley, 1986.

9. Lanes SF. The logic of causal inference in medicine. In this volume.

10. de Finetti B. Theory of Probability, Vol. 1. New York: Wiley, 1974.

11. Robins JM, Greenland S. The role of model selection in causal inference from nonexperimental data. Am J Epidemiol 1986;123:392–402.

12. Popper KR. The Logic of Scientific Discovery. Revised ed. New York: Harper and Row, 1968. Originally published as Logik der Forschung. Vienna: Springer, 1934.

13. Savage LJ. The Foundations of Statistics. New York: Wiley, 1954.

14. Popper KR. Quantum Theory and the Schism in Physics. Totowa, New Jersey: Rowman and Littlefield, 1982.

15. Harper WL, Hooker CA, eds. Foundations and Philosophy of Statistical Theories in the Physical Sciences (in three volumes). Dordrecht, Holland: D. Reidel, 1976.

16. Neutra RR, Greenland S, Friedman EA. The effect of fetal monitoring on cesarean rates. Obstet Gynecol 1980;55:175–180.

Inference in Epidemiology

Michael Jacobsen

Institute of Occupational Medicine
Edinburgh, Scotland.

. . . *the analysis of science—"the philosophy of science"—*
is threatening to become a fashion, a specialism.
K.R. Popper[1]

The Nature of Epidemiologic Inference

Epidemiologic inference is the process of drawing conclusions
about the distributions of health, of disease, and of their determinants, in groups of people. In most cases (it can be argued in
all cases) such inferences refer, explicitly or implicitly, to the *rela-*
tionships between those distributions. For instance, the smoking
patterns of people with and without lung cancer may provide
information justifying conclusions about the relationship between smoking and risks of developing lung cancer in the population from which the sample of individuals was taken. Or
consider any cross-sectional morbidity survey at one particular
industrial establishment. Implicit at least is the desire to compare
the prevalence rate of the condition being studied with the rate
in some other group that is characterized by a different type or
level of exposure to the hypothesized occupationally related de-

terminant. It is the *relationship* implicit in the joint distributions and the putative causal agent that is of interest.

Inferences of this kind, from particular observations to generalizations about the system from which the sample of observations has been taken, are usually described as inductive inferences. This nomenclature distinguishes such conclusions from those obtained using deductive arguments. A deductive conclusion is a particular statement about a particular event (or observation) that follows necessarily from a general axiomatic statement (or hypothesis) the truth of which is assumed for the sake of the argument.

Suppose for instance, as does Lanes[2] for the sake of his argument, that harboring a certain virus is a *necessary* and *sufficient* condition for the occurrence of the acquired immune deficiency syndrome (AIDS). It follows (from the assumption of sufficiency) that everyone who has the virus must have AIDS; and (necessarily) that anyone who does not have AIDS cannot be harboring the virus. A demonstration that a particular person without AIDS does not have the virus is certainly consistent with the theory, in that the theory has not been proven wrong. But, as Lanes notes, this single logical deduction, or even many such deductions about consistency, based on a large number of similar observations, tells us nothing about the etiology of AIDS or of any other disease. Note that aggregation of large numbers of *particular deductions* is not the same, by definition or conceptually, as making inductive generalizations from *particular observations*.

In the empirical sciences generally, and certainly in epidemiology, both methods of reasoning, inductive and deductive, are necessary and mutually supportive. But they are not the same. They do not obey the same rules. This fact is sometimes referred to as "the problem of induction."[1,2] One solution to the problem is to assert that "there is no such thing as induction;" "that induction is a myth;" "that sensible rules of induction do not exist."[3] (The quotations are from Popper, but he was certainly not the first philosopher to dismiss induction in this way. For instance, Bertrand Russell wrote in 1903: "I may as well say at once that I do not distinguish between inference and deduction.

What is called induction appears to me to be either disguised deduction or a mere method of making plausible guesses."[4]) Such assertions are unchallengeable if it is accepted, *a priori*, that the only sensible rules are deductive rules. But this would be a circular argument, since it merely restates the initial problem (the fact that the rules are not the same).

A better approach might be to compare inductive and deductive rules in epidemiology. We may then consider whether induction "can be applied without giving rise to inconsistencies; whether it helps us; and whether we really need it."[1]

"Why Bother?"

But first consider another question. Is it important (or even useful) for scientists to take an interest in these matters? Not really, says Schlesinger,[5] if they expect thereby to improve their experimental techniques or problem solving skills. On the contrary, say I. If the only advantage to be gained from debates of this kind is the satisfaction of individual scientists' curiosity about "understanding for the sake of understanding," if the intention is primarily to provide "mental exhilaration,"[5] then it would be difficult to justify devoting valuable time to these issues at professional meetings of epidemiologists. The reason why I believe it worthwhile for epidemiologists to discuss these abstractions is that I hope that it may help us to do our work more effectively. The better we are able to increase understanding about relationships between distributions of health, disease and their determinants, the easier it will be to prevent disease and promote health. And that, I like to think, is the aim of epidemiology. I take this aim as axiomatic, and the following comments are offered in that spirit.

Rules For Epidemiologic Inference

Here are some suggestions for "rules" ("principles," "criteria," "canons"—what you will) for making valid inferences in epidemiology.

1. Formulate as precisely as possible the question that you wish to answer in a way that is specific to the *distribution* of health and disease in *groups*.

2. Assemble data, of a kind and in a way, that are relevant to the study objectives.

3. Arrange the data in a way that will help to reveal patterns that are explicit or implicit in hypotheses contributing to the objectives.

4. Make predictions (from the sample of data) about the joint distributions of health, of disease and of factors that may influence them in the population(s) from which the data are drawn.

5. Examine critically the reliability of the predictions.

"Hold on" I hear someone say, "those may (or may not) be useful rules for conducting epidemiologic studies; but surely they are not rules for making epidemiologic *inferences*." My reply is that epidemiologic inferences are but a part of a wider (inductive) epidemiologic process. Of necessity, the rules for making the inferences must embrace rules for all other parts of the process. The (deductive) logic supporting this assertion is as follows. By hypothesis, epidemiologic generalizations are based on particular observations. Therefore the validity of epidemiologic inference depends necessarily on what kind of particular observations are made, how they are made, and how the data that they generate are arranged and analyzed. (Susser[6] disagrees: "Some authors include research method as a criterion for inference. . . . I do not consider it to be an attribute of an *association*.")

The following remarks may clarify how the proposed epidemiologic rules differ from conventional deductive rules. Figure 1 illustrates how the rules are linked in the continuous cycle of activity that constitutes epidemiology.

1. Objectives

The emphasis on *groups* and *distributions* in the rule for formulating epidemiologic objectives distinguishes them from objectives in clinical medicine. The latter refer to the problems of diseases

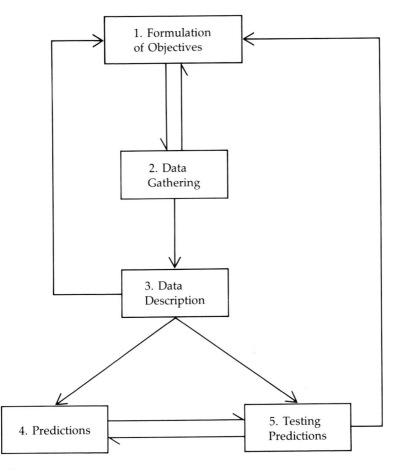

Figure 1
A model of the inductive process of epidemiology.

in individuals. The resolution of such problems will appeal more to deductive than to inductive reasoning: from assumed general medical knowledge to interpretation of the particular signs and symptoms that are presented by the patient.

2. Data gathering

Our textbooks, and many papers on design and methods in epidemiology, elaborate the rule that the data being assembled in an epidemiologic study must be relevant to the *epidemiologic* objective. No valid conclusions are possible from irrelevant data. One feature distinguishes epidemiologic data gathering very clearly from its analog in clinical medicine. The distributionally defined objectives in epidemiology require assembly of information not only about people with disease, but also about those who are healthy (for instance, "controls" in a case-control study). Acknowledgement of this principle (and its trivial corollary, that epidemiologic data gathering must not exclude information about those *with* disease) resolves Lanes'[2] illustration of what he calls "a paradox of induction." The supposed paradox arises only if rules 1 and 2 are ignored.

3. Data description

Again, the emphasis is on *relevance* to the objectives. Haphazard tabular or graphical arrangement may perhaps reveal some unexpected pattern that might suggest new research. But such serendipitous bonuses cannot, in general, lead to valid answers to previously defined epidemiologic questions.

Yet the pathway from elements 3 to 1 in Figure 1 reflects the fact that perusal of data gathered for any one specific purpose (e.g., regional morbidity data, to assist sensible allocation of limited national resources) may suggest an entirely new research question or hypothesis. The inductive process then continues at the point numbered 1 in the diagram.

4. Predictions

Epidemiologic predictions refer to the expected patterns of health and disease in groups, contingent on varying values of supposed determinants. Such predictions cannot be derived from an accumulation of separate clinical prognoses because individuals' responses to what are essentially identical stimuli are, in general, not predictable precisely. Yet application of rules 1 to 3 often reveals a pattern.

Unpredictability of individual outcomes, coupled with a regularity characteristic of the system comprising all possible outcomes, defines what statisticians call random systems. Quantitative predictions about random systems require statistical arguments. Three types of statistical predictions are recognized. One is in the form of statements about parameters that are likely to define the distributions of future observations (point estimates). Then there are statements about ranges of values that are likely to include the parameters that are being estimated (confidence intervals). Finally there are statements about the probability that results similar or even more extreme than those already observed may be expected to occur again, given appropriate assumptions (significance testing).

Informative analyses of epidemiologic data usually require all three kinds of predictions. Cox[7] also distinguishes usefully between three different kinds of applications for significance tests themselves: (i) calculation of p-values as indicators of consistency with some hypothesis; (ii) the use of significance tests as a form of decision rule; and (iii) their use in exploratory analyses, prior to formulating tentative conclusions.

Yet some authors[6,8] still seem to equate statistical inference with the calculation of p-values. It is not helpful to regard confidence intervals simply as surrogates for p-values ("to weigh probabilities of chance occurrence"[6]). Confidence intervals provide new information in their own right: they quantify the uncertainty associated with the predictions of the locations and shapes of distributions. Hypothesis testing, p-values and deductions about a singular alternative to a null hypothesis are not generally sufficient on their own.

A distinctive feature of statistical arguments is "to recognize explicitly that conclusions are uncertain and to attempt to measure that uncertainty."[7] This implies that epidemiological predictions do not have the characteristics of logically deduced syllogisms, irrespective of whether such deductions are expressed in words or in algebraic symbols.[9]

5. Testing predictions

Critical examination of predictions implied by epidemiological inferences is the central theme in Weed's contribution to this discussion;[10] and there appears to be unanimity about the importance of ensuring that hypotheses or theories must be testable, at least in principle, if they are to be classifiable legitimately as scientific hypotheses. But how, in practice, does one test an epidemiologically derived prediction? One way is to compare the predictions with results observed in similar studies elsewhere. If those studies were conducted in the past (and have been accepted as part of "pre-existing theory and knowledge") then this test would correspond, more or less, with Susser's coherence criterion.[6] But, as Susser points out, such coherence involves complex judgments and, when it is present, "usually does no more than afford a modest affirmation of a hypothesis." If new observational studies provide results affirmatively consistent with earlier predictions, then at least it can be said that the theory that underlies the prediction has not been falsified. Yet the most intuitively satisfying, quasi-experimental test of an epidemiologic prediction is to alter the distributions of hypothesized determinants of health and disease in real populations ("intervention"), to assess the results of the intervention (using rules 1 to 4), and to then compare the results of the intervention with the earlier predictions.

Some epidemiologists may recoil from the idea that decisions about public health policy (intervention) play a part in epidemiologic inference. But I am suggesting only that there is an important area of overlap between two distinct processes: one concerned with drawing valid conclusions from epidemiologic data, the other directed towards altering the future health-disease profile in the community (Figure 2). In that overlap area the two processes interact. In my opinion it is neither realistic nor helpful to ignore the reality of the interaction.[11] It is important to be clear however that although the processes interact, they are different.[2,12]

The Logico-Deductive Model

Logical deductions have been intertwined at various points in what I have called an inductive process of inference in epidemiology. This seems to be what Fisher had in mind when he suggested that "deductive arguments are, in fact, often only stages in an inductive process."[13] Others may argue that my repeated appeals to deductive logic simply confirm Russell's previously quoted claim, that what is called induction is often just disguised deduction.[4] Is this really so?

Figure 3 symbolizes the main features of the logico-deductive model for scientific discovery, as proposed by Popper[1] and as promoted by others.[2,8,10,14] There are some similarities with Figure 1, as might be expected if one accepts the idea that the inductive process of acquiring scientific knowledge involves frequent appeals to deductive argument. Yet the two models are different; the rules are *not* the same. Both diagrams reflect an acknowledgement that the growth of scientific knowledge is a continuing process. In Figure 3 this is represented by the loop from (va) back to (iii). A theory that survives an initial test is submitted to further tests of other predictions that it implies. The more tests that it survives, the bigger its contribution to knowledge. Just how much it contributes, i.e., what "degree of corroboration" for the hypothesis is obtained, is to be determined by the *sincerity* of the investigator's efforts to negate the hypothesis.[1] (This raises a problem for those, particularly psychologists,[14] who are convinced by Popper's dismissal of induction. How does one use logico-deductive principles to identify [let alone measure] *sincerity*?) But corroboration of an hypothesis is generally accorded a very subsidiary place in the model. The emphasis is always on tests that *refute* the hypothesis (element vi in Figure 3). Any one such falsified hypothesis reduces by just one the infinite number of alternative hypotheses that might be

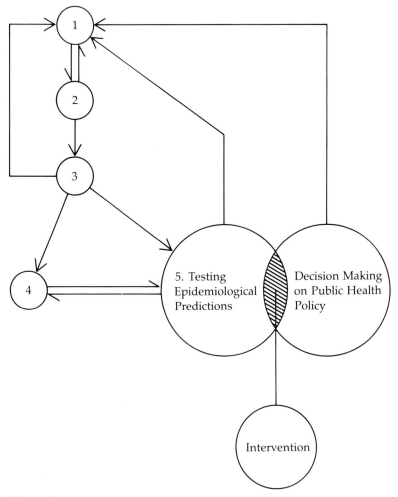

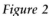

Figure 2
The interaction between epidemiology and decisions on public health.

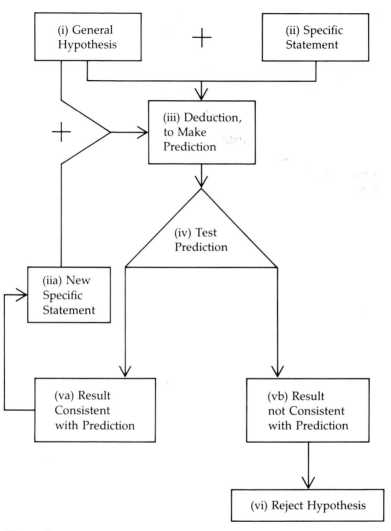

Figure 3
A logico-deductive (Popperian) model of scientific discovery.

proposed. And that, from the Popperian point of view, is essentially how scientific knowledge is advanced.

The reality of science is different. In practice, when a theory appears to be refuted, scientists ask themselves questions like: "Why was the theory refuted?" "How might it be improved?" "Was my method of testing (including the logic of the test) sound?" "Is there any useful information in the test results that will allow me to formulate a better theory?" etc. Surely such questions are part of the criticism that Weed[10] considers to be a reasonable philosophical guide to epidemiologic inference and to public health action. Yet these questions are all excluded specifically from the Popperian model of how knowledge grows. The process of generating ideas and objectives is outside the picture. It is, we are told, part of "the psychology of knowledge," and "it is irrelevant to the logical analysis of scientific knowledge."[1] A theory of knowledge thus divorced from the realities of scientific practice seems unsatisfactory to me.

Yet the important principle of testability (refutability) in science is recognized by all; and deductive logic is certainly an essential tool, not least in providing the theoretical framework of mathematical probability theory that is the basis for statistical inference. The inductive dynamics symbolized in Figure 1, and outlined above, accommodate these realities. The scheme is internally consistent and, I suggest, some such rules are both helpful and necessary in the practice of epidemiology. In particular, the inclusion of intervention as part of the process places epidemiologic inference into what I assumed axiomatically to be its proper perspective. This perspective is not merely "to learn something about the riddle of the world in which we live, and the riddle of man's knowledge of that world"[1]—it is difficult to reconcile even these objectives with the arbitrary *a priori* exclusion from the field of study of what Popper refers to as the "psychology of knowledge"—but to prevent disease and promote health.

References

1. Popper KR. *The Logic of Scientific Discovery*. Revised, 6th impression. London: Hutchinson, 1972. Originally published as *Logik der Forschung*. Vienna: Springer, 1934.

2. Lanes SF. The logic of causal inference in medicine. In this volume.

3. Popper K. *Unending Quest: an Intellectual Autobiography*. 2nd impression. Glasgow: Fontana/Collins, 1976.

4. Russell B. *The Principles of Mathematics*. 2nd ed., 8th impression. London: George Allen and Unwin, 1964:11.

5. Schlesinger G. Scientists and philosophy. In this volume.

6. Susser M. Falsification, verification and causal inference in epidemiology: reconsideration in the light of Sir Karl Popper's philosophy. In this volume.

7. Cox DR. Theory and general principle in statistics. J R Stat Soc A 1981;144:289–294.

8. Buck C. Popper's philosophy for epidemiologists. Int J Epidemiol 1975;4:159–168.

9. Jacobsen M. Against Popperized epidemiology. Int J Epidemiol 1976;5:9–11.

10. Weed DL. Causal criteria and Popperian refutation. In this volume.

11. Jacobsen M. Scientists and safety. New Scientist 1977;75:40–41.

12. Jacobsen M. Occupational health risk assessment. In: Hester RE, ed. *Industry and the Environment in Perspective*. Special Publication No. 46, London: Royal Society of Chemistry, 1983:179–189.

13. Fisher RA. *Statistical Methods and Scientific Inference*. Revised, 2nd ed. Edinburgh: Oliver and Boyd, 1959:109.

14. Eysenck HJ. Who needs a random sample? Bull Br Psychol Soc 1975;28:196–198.

Epidemiologic Inference

Darwin R. Labarthe and Reuel A. Stallones

The EpiCenter
School of Public Health
The University of Texas Health Science Center
Houston, Texas

Concepts of Causation: *Whatever constructs we may devise must be understood to represent our biased views of what a representation of reality should be. Because it is not the reality, the value of the model depends upon its utility, and utility depends upon the purpose for which the model is used. . . . An approach that holds promise is to consider the interdependence of a number of diseases, characteristics of individuals, and environmental and social variables as elements in a constellation which is n-dimensional, and within which directed pathways are incidental to the complex as a whole.*
R.A. Stallones[1]

The passage cited above was, and is, intended to convey a view of epidemiology as being both virtually universal and quite particular in scope, both highly theoretical and eminently pragmatic in concept, and capable of both grandeur and circumspection in attitude. We approach the subject of epidemiologic inference and the question of its philosophical legitimacy from this viewpoint.

Two issues need attention as background. The first concerns "epidemiologic inference," a term that may be variously understood. To illustrate the usage that antedates the present symposium may provide a helpful perspective. The second is whether, if we had a problem of epidemiologic inference, the philosophy of science should be expected to offer a ready solution. Both of these questions are basic to the papers assembled here.

From the viewpoint suggested above, and with the background to be provided, we will then discuss briefly the three issues that seem central to the four papers under discussion. They are the following:

(1) Is Hill the/a villain?

(2) Is Popper the/a hero? and

(3) How do the answers to (1) and (2) depend on one's view of epidemiology?

Epidemiologic Inference and Philosophy

A half-century ago, Wade Hampton Frost characterized epidemiology as:

> . . . something more than the total of its established facts. It includes their orderly arrangement into *chains of inference* which extend more or less beyond the bounds of direct observation. Such of those chains as are well and truly laid guide investigation to the facts of the future; those that are ill made fetter progress. But it is not easy, when divergent theories are presented, to distinguish immediately between those which are sound and those which are merely plausible.[2] (emphasis added)

This passage, familiar to all students of epidemiology, has immediate as well as historical relevance, as demonstrated by the papers presented in this symposium. Perhaps less familiar, but no less relevant, is Frost's further characterization,

> . . . epidemiology is essentially an inductive science, concerned not merely with describing the distribution of disease, but equally or more with fitting it into a consistent philosophy.[3]

His emphasis here is on that reasoning that proceeds from the particular to the general, from observations to theories. But the further problems of evaluating competing theories and extending observations under the guidance of accepted ones are also clearly identified in the first of these passages from Frost.

In another setting, not consciously epidemiologic, Platt uses the term "strong inference" to denote the following procedure:

(1) Devising alternative hypotheses;

(2) Devising a crucial experiment (or several of them), with alternative possible outcomes, each of which will, as nearly as possible, exclude one or more of the hypotheses;

(3) Carrying out the experiment so as to get a clean result;

(1') Recycling the procedure, making subhypotheses or sequential hypotheses to refine the possibilities that remain; and so on.[4]

If for "crucial experiment" we substitute "rigorous epidemiologic investigation," the procedure becomes applicable in principle in epidemiology as well as in biophysics and the other fields that were Platt's intended target. Of course, not all of epidemiologic research could be characterized in this way. But studies beginning from an explicit hypothesis and designed to test it, especially with prior specification of alternatives, would surely qualify. This approach is a commonly cited classroom ideal.

Interestingly, Platt refers to this process as "inductive inference" but later cites Popper in discussing how hypotheses are devised and tested. In so doing, Platt clearly embraces the view that science advances by the same process of formulation and falsification of hypotheses that Popper discusses as the "hypothetical-deductive method."[5] If, therefore, strong inference is importantly deductive inference, and if Frost's view demonstrates the necessary place of inductive inference in epidemiology, then epidemiologists should be wary of any philosophical argument too narrow to accommodate both.

These general considerations are in keeping with the broader views of epidemiology suggested in our opening comments. To our reading, "epidemiologic inference" as referred to in this symposium is sometimes, but not consistently, much stricter in intent and more selective in its reference to specific aspects of epidemiologic thinking. The importance of this fact for the possibility of drawing an overall conclusion will become apparent.

If we cast our attention further toward philosophy, we find that uncertainty and controversy are not the sole province of epidemiology. Philosophy is also alive. Philosophical matters thought incontrovertible by the novice can be seen for their substantial complexity on even a casual examination. Anyone who doubts this will be enlightened by reading such pieces as "Why" or "Reasons and Causes" in *The Encyclopedia of Philosophy*.[6] The contributors to this symposium provide supporting evidence that the philosophy of science may be no freer of controversy, or at least diversity, than is epidemiology.

We are now in a position to test the hypothesis that there are problems about epidemiologic inference for which the philosophers have the needed solution.

Issues Raised by the Symposium

(1) Is Hill the/a villain?
Sir Austin Bradford Hill is occasionally held liable for a doctrinaire codification of rules for causal inference the application of which lacks logic, rigor and objectivity. His place in the development of causal thinking in epidemiology deserves to be better understood.

First, his noteworthy address, "The Environment and Disease: Association or Causation?," presented and published in 1965, had important antecedents.[7] For example, special concerns about causation of chronic diseases were addressed quite explicitly in a series of three articles appearing in the *Journal of Chronic Diseases* in 1959 and 1960.[8,9,10] Here Yerushalmy and Palmer, then Lilienfeld, and then Sartwell discussed the merits and limitations of Koch's postulates for establishing causality in non-infectious diseases. In content, if not in actual development (Hill does not cite Sartwell), Hill's list includes and supplements that of Sartwell published 5 years earlier. Much earlier, some of the qualities of epidemiologic evidence that may tend to lend conviction concerning causation had been given less formally by Frost, in discussing Snow's observations on cholera.[2] Thus Hill's contribution had readily identifiable antecedents and was not unique in either its focus or its approach.

Second, Hill's presentation was anything but dogmatic. In fact, even the word "criteria," now commonly applied to the set of interpretive guidelines as he proposed them or as later modified, does not appear in his text. Rather, he cited as a "consideration," "characteristic," or "feature" of the evidence each of the qualities identified in his list. He wrote on this point as follows:

> Here then are nine different viewpoints from all of which we should study association before we cry causation. What I do not believe—and this has been suggested—is that we can usefully lay down some hard-and-fast rules of evidence that *must* be obeyed before we accept cause and effect. None of my nine viewpoints can bring indisputable evidence for or against the cause-and-effect hypothesis and none can be required as a *sine qua non*. What they can do, with greater or less strength, is to help us to make up our minds on the fundamental question—is there any other way of explaining the set of facts before us, is there any other answer equally, or more, likely than cause and effect?[7]

Hill was proposing an approach to the interpretation of evidence that is closely analogous to that advocated by Platt for its collection: the consideration of alternative hypotheses, here of causal vs. other explanations of an association, and an attempt at refutation of the alternatives by some systematic procedure. That the proposed procedure has sometimes (often?) been insufficient to assure uniformity of interpretation by all interested parties should pose no disillusionment. Nor should this circumstance be taken to discredit the contributions of Hill and others to the general problem. Even if wholly satisfactory themselves, the use of such "viewpoints" as Hill's is only one phase of the overall process of evaluating and interpreting epidemiologic evidence. For example, the Burch-Lilienfeld-Burch exchange (in which the application of the criteria in the Surgeon General's Report of 1982 was alternately attacked and defended) illustrates fundamental differences in the judgments—and judgments they are, notwithstanding protestations to the contrary by Burch—concerning the admissibility of particular observations into evidence, as well as other difficulties not intrinsic to the procedure itself.[11,12,13]

The four writers in this symposium diverge sharply on the

subject of Hill and the "criteria" attributed to him. Weed claims that the criteria are inadequate as rules for making causal inferences, chiefly on grounds of their failure to conform with canons of Popperian refutation, as he interprets these. He proposes replacement of the criteria by his two candidates, "predictability" and "testability," which he then curiously justifies by reason of their close congruence with the original criteria of Hill (excepting that of "analogy," which he wholly rejects). In closing, Weed ventures that "some of Hill's original criteria will continue to provide epidemiologists with a basis for inference." In some instances, he implies, this circumstance will not be inappropriate.

Susser maintains that Hill's criteria are worthy of improvement but, by contrast with Weed, suggests more of an evolutionary than a revolutionary approach. His revised list is as follows:

Probability
Time order

Direction
{
Strength
Specificity
Consistency
Predictive performance
Coherence
}

In conventional terms, "probability" has to do with the question whether an association is evident at all, prior to the application of any procedure for its interpretation. "Direction," or "whether X *leads to* Y," seems only to serve to set apart from the remaining criteria what he terms "time order," which is thereby invested with a special hierarchical pre-eminence. Susser's introduction of "predictive performance" is at first appealing but taken literally risks becoming a *reductio ad infernum*: It poses the question whether a theory or hypothesis has successfully predicted offspring that are verified (or not falsified) by the test of observation; but how could one decide on the success of the prediction except by applying to the new observations the whole set of the criteria that contain this one?; and so on. Perhaps an occasion for fuller explication and illustration will be more persuasive of the improvement.

Lanes expresses intolerance for the vagueness of language about causality in epidemiology (and stops far short of an "exhaustive expose"), which sorry state he attributes mainly to our confusion ("uncertainty") about the interpretation of causal theories. The criteria of Hill and others he totally rejects as a mere device for codifying "beliefs." They [the criteria] "survive only on the faith of their followers; they have no logical foundation." Clearly we have room for further exploration, if not a narrowing, of differences among the present philosophers.

Schlesinger moves us nowhere on this particular issue, however. Having reserved until his final paragraph any mention of epidemiology, he has missed the opportunity to discuss such specifically epidemiologic matters as criteria for interpretation of evidence. He has other things to say, and his contributions lie elsewhere.

(2) Is Popper the/a hero?
Most epidemiologists' affairs with Popper probably began with his introduction by Carol Buck, 10 years ago.[14] As with any new acquaintance, he was received and understood variously.[15,16,17] As noted above, Platt had cited Popper earlier and substantially embraced his view that "science advances only by disproofs."[4] Platt went further:

The difficulty is that disproof is a hard doctrine. If you have a hypothesis and I have another hypothesis, evidently one of them must be eliminated. The scientist seems to have no choice but to be either soft-headed or disputatious. Perhaps this is why so many tend to resist the strong analytical approach—and why some great scientists are so disputatious.

(One is reminded of those of our students who, aspiring to greatness, acquire first the disputatiousness described; we may often serve as better models of the intermediate than of the long-range goal.)

Among the four writers here, all give some attention to Popper, but again in quite divergent ways. For Weed, as already discussed, Popper provides the logical foundation for rewriting Hill's criteria. Susser is less deferential and points to certain limitations in the application of Popper's approach to epidemiology. He rejects Popper's exclusive use of deduction, in recognition of the pragmatic value of induction from available observations. He also rejects what is attributed to Popper as a view of "asymmetry" between falsification and verification, contending that falsification of hypotheses or theories is no less fallible than is their verification. This view calls attention to an important problem that warrants further consideration, as will be noted below.

For Lanes, Popper's authority is absolute. Lanes insists on refutation but fails to recognize, as Platt anticipates and as Susser implies, that refutation may entail difficulties of its own. How, for example, is refutation accomplished? Are the procedures for refuting one or another causal hypothesis qualitatively distinct from those for refuting alternative, non-causal hypotheses? Does recourse to the exclusively Popperian view really solve the problem, or does it simply beg the question?

Schlesinger is silent on Popper, except to cite a "delightfully witty, devastating criticism" that features Popper as one of "the four contemporary irrationalists" (with Lakatos, Kuhn and Feyerabend). Schlesinger appears to enjoy, and perhaps welcome, the devastation.

As with their positions on Hill, the four present writers are far apart concerning Popper. Having abandoned any expectation of an immediate philosophical resolution of epidemiologic problems, we may yet gain something from considering the basis for these striking differences.

(3) How do the answers to (1) and (2) depend on one's view of epidemiology?

The final thread that can be woven through the four papers collected here represents the concepts of epidemiology that the writers express or imply. From the perspective we suggested in opening this discussion, a duality of theory and practice, or of explanation and prevention, is intrinsic to epidemiology. Without sound theory, epidemiologic practice may be misguided and frivolous; without practical application, epidemiologic theory may be sterile and fruitless. The present papers, taken together, chasten the expectation that epidemiologic theory and practice can presently, if ever, be reduced to a single, purely and wholly logical basis. They suggest instead that the logic of scientific advancement and the rationale for practical decision making are better regarded as distinct, though closely related. From this viewpoint, the divergence of opinions of the first two questions becomes easily understood. Hypothesis: An exclusive reliance on formal logic is advocated most strictly where the practical domain of epidemiology is recognized least. Do the observations fit the prediction?

Among the four writers, the pattern is as follows: Weed dismisses what he calls "causal action" as falling beyond the pale of logic, but he at least acknowledges it; recall that, although invoking Popper to revolutionize Hill's criteria, Weed does also leave some room for those criteria (at least as newly-interpreted) even if judged to have limited utility. Susser is not explicit concerning practical applications, but we are disposed to believe that this is so obvious in his view that its mention is superfluous; he proposes to strengthen the criteria, based in part on his revisions of the Popperian approach. Lanes is extreme in all respects, that is, in the absolutism of Popper, the absolute rejection of criteria such as Hill's, and the absolute segregation of science from practice. Finally, Schlesinger is in these respects essentially mute: He has instead sought to disabuse us against taking philosophers at face value; to extoll the generosity of nature in revealing fundamental laws in an indulgent way; and to encourage epidemiologists to emulate those successful in other fields in order to establish such laws in the health sciences. The universe, he concludes poetically, is "user friendly."

We observe that the various predispositions concerning practical epidemiology, among only these three writers who betray them, seem strongly related to their attitudes toward criteria (Hill and others) and toward deductive logic (Popper). This pattern suggests that a separation of issues, as between the advancement of knowledge and the improvement of practice, would reduce the complexity of our early gropings in this business—much as Schlesinger characterizes the humbler beginnings in several areas of science. A useful step in advancing future explorations of philosophy and epidemiology would be to examine theory and practice both independently and as they intersect. It appears that the issues, the attitudes, and the proposals for resolution would be different in each of the two areas; their intersections in all three respects would be something to contemplate.

Conclusions

(1) There is variation among views of epidemiology.

(2) There is variation among views of philosophy.

(3) The evidence of this symposium suggests a strong interdependence between (1) and (2), within that tiny proportion of the population having views of both.

(4) Equally evident is that criteria are needed for the interpretation of philosophical advice. To judge those criteria, it would seem that epidemiologists are on their own.

References

1. Stallones RA. To advance epidemiology. Ann Rev Public Health 1980;1:69–82.

2. Frost WH. *Introducton to Snow on Cholera; Being a Reprint of Two Papers by John Snow, MD.* New York: The Commonwealth Fund, 1936.

3. Maxcy KF, ed. *Papers of Wade Hampton Frost, MD. A Contribution to Epidemiologic Method.* New York: Arno Press, 1977.

4. Platt JR. Strong inference. Science 1964;146:347–353.

5. Popper KR. The hypothetical-deductive method and the unity of social and natural science. In: *Karl R. Popper. The Poverty of Historicism.* New York: Harper and Row, 1961.

6. Edwards P, ed. *The Encyclopedia of Philosophy.* New York: The MacMillan Company and the Free Press, 1967.

7. Hill AB. The environment and disease: association or causation? Proc Roy Soc Med 1965;58:295–300.

8. Yerushalmy J, Palmer CE. On the methodology of investigations of etiologic factors in chronic diseases. J Chronic Dis 1959;10:27–40.

9. Lilienfeld AM. "On the methodology of investigations of etiologic factors in chronic diseases." Some comments. J Chronic Dis 1959;10:41–46.

10. Sartwell PE. "On the methodology of investigations of etiologic factors in chronic diseases." Further comments. J Chronic Dis 1959;11:61–63.

11. Burch PRJ. The Surgeon General's "Epidemiologic criteria for causality." A critique. J Chronic Dis 1983;36:821–836.

12. Lilienfeld AM. The Surgeon General's "Epidemiologic criteria for causality." A criticism of Burch's critique. J Chronic Dis 1983;36:837–845.

13. Burch PRJ. The Surgeon General's "Epidemiologic criteria for causality." Reply to Lilienfeld [Letter]. J Chronic Dis 1984;37:148–156.

14. Buck C. Popper's philosophy for epidemiologists. Int J Epidemiol 1975;4:159–168.

15. Davies MA. Comments on "Popper's philosophy for epidemiologists." Comment one. Int J Epidemiol 1975;4:169–171.

16. Smith A. Comments on "Popper's philosophy for epidemiologists." Comment two. Int J Epidemiol 1975;4:169–171.

17. Jacobsen M. Against Popperized epidemiology. Int J Epidemiol 1976;5:9–11.

Refutation in Epidemiology: Why Else Not?

Malcolm Maclure

Department of Epidemiology
Harvard School of Public Health
Boston, Massachusetts

The invitation to comment on four different views of the philosophy of science in epidemiology provides a unique opportunity to test and to further develop the hypothesis that refutation of competing explanations is the essence of the scientific method in epidemiology. I propose to test it by critically examining the alternative or contrary opinions expressed by Schlesinger and Susser, and seeing whether they can be refuted. I propose to develop the hypothesis further by scrutinizing the refutationist perspectives of Weed and Lanes for weaknesses or inconsistencies.

I begin my commentary with Schlesinger's paper since he raises the question of whether your reading this book has any practical benefit. He starts by writing "Is it important for a scientist to take an interest in the philosophy of science? Not very much if thereby he expects to improve his experimental technique or problem solving skills." Yet in his final paragraph, he concludes that one of the reasons a scientist should be interested in philosophy is "A thorough investigation of the various aspects of reality that have facilitated our rapid understanding of nature's laws may have a profound impact on the scientist's practical conduct." This contradiction makes his paper rather difficult to digest.

He also appears to contradict himself by seeming to accept Stove's "devastating criticism" of refutationists Popper, Lakatos, Kuhn and Feyerabend, while elsewhere arguing that philosophy is in "a deplorable state of affairs" because the metaphysical hypotheses of philosophy are less testable than the hypotheses of natural sciences. Throughout his article he makes statements that indicate the importance he attaches to deductive refutation as a means of keeping philosophy rooted in reality:

The method of counterexamples [refutation] is of course widely practiced in philosophical polemics, but with radically less firm results than in mathematics. . . . Much of mathematics has practical applications and hence invalid arguments can be detected [i.e., hypotheses refuted] in those cases in ultimately the same way as in the physical sciences.

Our discipline [philosophy] is not entirely without its defenses. . . . [C]ommon sense—that has been said to be the knack for seeing things as they are—can provide a mechanism for the rejection [refutation] of undesirable elements.

Theses that flagrantly misrepresent reality are likely to be discredited [refuted]. . . .

There is a third more subtle contradiction. On the one hand, he criticizes the idea that our observations are conditioned by our theories. On the other hand, he remarks how fortunate it was that the Greeks had acquainted us with ellipses, hyperbolas, and parabolas because (he implies) this helped us to recognize the trajectories of planets, comets, and other objects whose paths are curved by gravitational forces.

Although Schlesinger's article is pleasantly stimulating, one need not read past the first paragraph to glean the essence of his argument and his error. He writes "just as an acquaintance with the theory of mechanics is virtually useless in facilitating the performance of the high-wire artist, so the study of philosophy is unlikely to contribute much to a scientist's competence." This view is refuted by the well-documented examples of modern athletes and coaches using knowledge of the principles of mechanics and physiology to improve their performances.

Susser's article provides a further refutation of Schlesinger's assertion that philosophizing cannot improve a scientist's problem-solving skills. By reviewing and further developing Hill's criteria for causal inference, Susser leads the reader to think more deeply about the ingredients of the process of drawing conclusions from data. Inference is an important problem-solving skill that distinguishes the experienced epidemiologist from the naive.

It is nice to see Susser stress the importance of the refutationist approach in inference and conclude, "We may follow Popper to the extent of claiming somewhat greater decisiveness for falsification than affirmation. . . ." So long as Susser's readers are convinced of the importance of continually hypothesizing alternative explanations and seeking evidence that discriminates among the alternatives, then I am sympathetic. I worry, however, that his view of verification and falsification as symmetric provides uncritical researchers with excuses for bolstering their conclusions and slackening their attention to alternative explanations.

Susser is more of a refutationist than he claims. He singles out specificity-in-the-cause, strength of association and consistency as the criteria that contribute greatest "support" to a causal hypothesis. Yet what is specificity-in-the-cause? It is the absence of (i.e., refutation of) alternative causes. As concerns the strength of association, Susser himself writes, "the stronger the relationship, the less a confounding variable capable of explaining the association is likely to exist." In other words, a strong association is supportive insofar as it refutes confounders. Thus, if an association is strong but there are many possible alternative explanations (e.g., a crude association between a disease and a specific nutrient in the diet, such as carotene), then the strength of the association is less supportive because it is less successful at refuting the alternatives (e.g., there are many possible positive and negative confounders that could explain the association with carotene). Finally, we turn to consistency, which Susser says "is the most powerful verification available." Again, however, the reason it is powerful is because it amounts to refutation of sundry alternative explanations. In Susser's words, "Consistency is present if the result is not dislodged in the face of diversity in times, places, circumstances, and people, as well as of research design." In other words, characteristics of the particular times, places, circumstances, people, and designs of the early studies that might have been alternative explanations for the association when it was first seen are refuted by later studies in which these characteristics are absent and yet the association prevails.

Weed also writes about Hill's criteria for causal inference, but more critically. Hill was somewhat vague about what he meant by causation and Weed explores the ramifications of being more precise. Specifying alternative, more precisely formulated concepts of causation, Weed asks to what extent Hill's criteria follow logically from each particular definition of causation. He concludes that only a few of the criteria are deducible if, by "cause," we mean sufficient cause or component cause as defined in epidemiologic terms. He asserts, however, that more of the criteria are directly deducible (i.e., are logical manifestations of our definition of causation) if we adopt a more mechanistic model of causation—"a cause acting in a multistage disease process."

Having criticized Hill's criteria as inadequate, Weed proposes two alternative criteria: predictability and testability. His goal is to show that Hill's criteria are explained by fewer, more fundamental criteria. This is a laudable goal. It is always nice to discover that several diverse phenomena are manifestations of a singular underlying phenomenon. (For example, it is helpful to appreciate that the rules for detecting confounding in stratified analyses or logistic models, in case-control studies or in follow-up studies, all follow logically from a single definition of a confounder as an alternative cause of disease associated with the exposure of interest.) Unfortunately, it is not clear to me that he succeeds. Weed's (or should I say Popper's) criteria of predictability and testability are characteristics of scientific *hypotheses* whereas Hill's criteria are characteristics of *data* (either aspects of an observed association or types of indirect evidence). So I cannot see how the former can replace the latter.

Weed states that his article is a response to my suggestion that Hill's criteria should be interpreted as criteria for refuting rather than demonstrating causal hypotheses. I am glad to have stimulated a response of any kind but I had in mind something different from Weed's approach. I can best explain by use of examples:

(a) *Strength of Association*: The repeatedly observed negative association between moderate alcohol intake and cardiovascular disease (CVD) tends to refute the hypothesis that moderate alcohol intake causes cardiovascular disease. On the other hand, a strong positive association between nicotine and CVD does not prove that nicotine is a risk factor because it is wholly confounded by other ingredients of tobacco smoke.

(b) *Consistency*: The frequent inability to reproduce the occasionally observed association between type A personality and CVD tends to refute the causal hypothesis. On the other hand, the consistently observed association between obesity and CVD does not rule out the possibility that both are outcomes of shared causes rather than the former being a cause of the latter.

(c) *Specificity*: An association between a particular plasma lipid fraction and CVD is not a specific association insofar as there are many other biochemical parameters correlated with CVD. The lack of specificity tends to refute a causal interpretation of any one association.

(d) *Temporality*: If a physiologic abnormality, such as hypertension, originates only after the development of diabetes, this sequence refutes the hypothesis that hypertension caused the diabetes. By contrast, the precedence of diabetes by increased hypertension does not confirm an etiologic relation between the two.

(e) *Biologic Gradient*: A J-shape in the curve of all-cause mortality when plotted against percent of ideal weight raises a flag of skepticism. The lack of a linear relation is a suggestion that there may be some confounding. Two likely explanations come to mind: people at the low end of the body-weight scale are thinner because they smoke more or because they have diseases that contribute to their increased mortality. In short, departures from expected biologic gradients provide evidence against causation. The converse does not necessarily hold. A smooth "dose-response" relation between reduced calorie intake and obesity does not support the hypothesis that obesity is caused by undereating. The gradient is a manifestation of confounding by physical activity.

(f) *Plausibility*: The so-called constitutional theory that a genetic characteristic predisposes some people to take up smoking and to quit smoking more easily, while at the same time predisposing them to CVD and cancer by separate mechanisms, is hard to accept. Why? Because evidence from many different disciplines corroborates a model of human physiology that is so complex, we can be pretty sure that a multitude of modifiers and independent factors would contribute substantial "noise" to the convoluted causal chain hypothesized by the constitutional theory.

Relative risks of 2 to 10 argue for a much simpler, more direct causal chain. The constitutional theory is refuted because it is implausible. On the other hand, the plausibility of innumerable refuted theories, from the "bad air" theory of malaria to the chemical toxin theory of Legionnaire's disease, did not contribute support to them after the unexpected discoveries of the microorganisms responsible for these diseases.

(g) *Experimental Evidence*: A double-blind randomized trial of aspirin as a preventive of myocardial infarction is the best way to test that hypothesis because randomization eliminates selection bias and minimizes confounding, while blinding eliminates observation bias. Alternative explanations are thereby refuted and the hypothesis is tested cleanly. Failure to demonstrate the association in *any* experimental animal model tends to refute a hypothesis whereas finding an association in experiments with a particular species of rodent or mammal does not provide much support for the hypothesis as applied to humans.

(h) *Analogy*: Analogy is mainly useful as a tool for refutation: we draw heavily on analogies when we hypothesize confounding by the "healthy worker effect" or bias in selection of a hospital control group.

(i) *Coherence*: Coherence means all the pieces fit together in a harmonious chorus. If 10 new voices are added to the chorus, 9 harmonious and 1 dissonant, the dissonant voice rightfully grabs more attention. Nine replications of the association between fat intake and CVD carry less weight than the observation of lower

CVD among Eskimos whose diets are rich in fat. Pound for pound, an incoherent piece of evidence is more influential than a coherent piece.

Hill's criteria are therefore a useful set of tests to which causal hypotheses should be submitted, but they serve our purposes best if we are fully cognizant that they contribute only insofar as they refute the causal hypothesis or competing explanations.

Lanes' article is the most consonant with my own views. I would make only two points. My first concerns a missed opportunity in his use of AIDS as an example. He writes, "the theory that a certain virus is a necessary cause of AIDS can be refuted only by observing an AIDS patient who does not harbor the virus." Some readers will surely ask "What about the seronegative cases?" Lanes could have used this example to illustrate how refutation is not final because it is conditional upon the theories inherent in any contradictory observation. Even after HTLV-III/LAV had been discovered, it was occasionally difficult to detect antibodies to the virus in full-blown AIDS patients. There were therefore two conflicting hypotheses, one of which had to be refuted: (a) HTLV-III/LAV is a necessary cause of AIDS, or (b) inability to detect antibodies to the virus in an AIDS patient means he was never exposed to HTLV-III/LAV. The latter hypothesis was eventually refuted and consequently, the former was corroborated.

Second, Lanes' discussion of the relation of science and policymaking would have been clearer to the reader if he had explained that scientists formulate and test (by refutation) *etiologic* hypotheses whereas policymakers formulate and test (by implementation and criticism) *ethical* hypotheses. Both science and enlightened policymaking occur against a background of untested beliefs about causation and uncritical convictions about what should be done. Both scientific knowledge (etiologic theories) and civilized policy (ethical theories) advance through the process of refutation. The difference is that scientists are concerned with the pursuit of Truth whereas policymakers must pursue both Truth and Value. Lanes draws attention to this but implies that the methodology of good policymaking and good science are quite different. I think the similarities are striking.

I wish to conclude my commentary by asserting an ethical hypothesis: I believe epidemiologists should recognize that refutation is the underpinning of good epidemiologic science. The alternatives are induction, intuition or conventions. These alternatives are evidently inadequate. Guided by intuition and convention, a lot of shoddy epidemiology gets sent to publishers and some of it passes peer review and gets printed. Why? Refutation is counter-intuitive and many conventions in epidemiology are justified by verificationist arguments. I think the quality of research, writing and reviewing would be improved if the central place of refutation were more widely appreciated. The common thread running through bad studies, whether their weakness is in the design, conduct, analysis or interpretation, is insufficient attention to alternative explanations. The take-home message is: We should always ask "Why else?" and then try to show "Why not."

The Truth, the Whole Truth, and Nothing but the Truth?

Neil McIntyre

Academic Department of Medicine,
Royal Free Hospital and School of Medicine,
London, England

I was flattered to be asked to comment on these four papers. I am neither an epidemiologist nor a philosopher. I write as a clinical academic whose work involves patient care and the teaching of medical students, as well as clinical and biomedical research. I admit to being a follower of Sir Karl Popper because I believe that his writings have much to offer medical scientists and teachers, and I was pleased to see how they have stimulated three of the authors of the accompanying papers.

My belief in the usefulness of some of Popper's work for the practicing scientist may explain my dissatisfaction with Schlesinger's paper on "Scientists and Philosophy," which begins with the statement that "the study of philosophy is unlikely to contribute much to a scientist's performance." This may be true of philosophy in general and of much of the published work on the philosophy of science, but I do not believe it is true for the study of Popper's ideas. His arguments against inductionism, his emphasis on a hypothetico-deductive approach, and his suggestion that the best way to test a hypothesis is to attempt to show that it is false all appear to me to have important practical implications for scientists who accept them, as the arguments must affect their experimental approach. Therefore, I found it irritating that Schlesinger's only comment on Popper implied that he is largely a popularizer of his own ideas.

I had not previously read the article in *Encounter* to which Schlesinger refers. Stove makes disparaging remarks about Popper.[1] I was not suprised to find that Popper's ideas were distorted; like other writers he has often been subjected to misrepresentation of his views, often by people who do not appear to have read what he has written. What did surprise me was that Stove impugned the motives underlying Popper's work. I don't know whether he wrote tongue in cheek, as suggested by his title "Karl Popper and the Jazz Age;" what I do know is that his article is not based on the rational and critical approach to argument that is repeatedly advocated by Popper. I suggest that readers should judge Popper's work for themselves, by reading what he has actually written.[2,3,4] I am sure they will find it a rewarding experience.

Causal Criteria and Popperian Refutation

In general I agree with many of Weed's comments. Clearly epidemiologic hypotheses should allow predictions to be made and these predictions should be testable, at least in theory. I say "at least in theory" because in practice it is sometimes impossible to test a hypothesis if the necessary facilities and methods are not available.

I step on thin ice in entering an argument about epidemiologic methods and principles. Nevertheless, it appears to me that the "Popperian" alternatives to Hill's criteria are not really alternatives. Hill's criteria relate to the nature of the relation between the event and the proposed cause, while predictability and testability relate to the nature of the hypothesis. Surely the recognition that one or more of Hill's criteria appear to be satisfied is a sound basis for formulating a hypothesis about a causal relation; the hypothesis allows predictions to be made that can then be tested. If many of Hill's criteria appear to have been satisfied then it seems likely that a very reasonable hypothesis can be formulated. But even if all of them are satisfied, it does not mean that the resulting hypothesis will turn out to be true. Furthermore, a better hypothesis may be formulated (in the sense that it will withstand subsequent attempts at falsification) even if it started from a situation where none of Hill's criteria had been met (though it would then be difficult to account for the origin of the hypothesis—other than as a flash of epidemiologic inspiration!). These points are in fact implicit in the last few paragraphs of Weed's paper.

I was disappointed that Weed did not attempt to answer his own question "How then can we make reasonable decisions to act, in the face of this certain uncertainty?" It is sometimes suggested that Popper's insistence on the inevitable incompleteness of knowledge makes it difficult to act on available information (as implied in the question above). Popper's position is not that we should take no action but rather that we should not *rely* on the underlying theory (in the sense of accepting it to be the truth). If action is needed then,

we should prefer the best tested theory as the basis of action. The best tested theory is the one which, in the light of the critical discussion, appears to be the best so far.[5]

It is, of course, important that we should review the results of our action; by so doing we test the hypothesis and demonstrate implicitly our unwillingness to "rely" on the theory.

The Logic of Causal Inference in Medicine

I am in almost complete agreement with the views expressed in Lanes' article "The Logic of Causal Inference in Medicine." I would point out one dilemma. In the first paragraph of section III he considers the theory "that exposure to a certain virus is a necessary cause of AIDS." He then states that the details of the theory imply that every AIDS patient harbors the virus, and that the theory also implies that people who do not harbor the virus do not have AIDS. However, a person harboring the virus does not necessarily have AIDS. The details missing from Lanes' brief comments would presumably include the criteria on which the diagnosis of AIDS can be made; if the presence of the virus is considered an essential criterion then the theory cannot be refuted and the "detailed theory" would not be a scientific statement, at least as far as the causal nature of the relation is concerned.

Based on these considerations, one might question whether Popper's scientific views can be applied to the problem of clinical diagnosis. Certainly it is possible to refute diagnostic hypotheses by the performance of appropriate tests (though this is a far from perfect process). Is it possible to confirm diagnoses with certainty? Although it may be difficult in practice the answer in theory must be "yes," because diagnosis is essentially a process of allocating a patient to a diagnostic class. When we use the name of a disease or syndrome for the purpose of classification we are not labelling something that exists in its own right; we are using a definition. As Popper has pointed out, good definitions in science should be read from right to left and not from left to right. The sentence "A di-neutron is an unstable system comprising two neutrons" is the scientist's answer to the question "what shall we call an unstable system comprising two neutrons"—not an answer to the question "what is a di-neutron?" The word "di-neutron" is a handy substitute for a long description, but no information about physics is to be gained from analyzing it.[6]

The relevance for diagnosis is obvious. We make a diagnosis of "diabetes mellitus" or "myocardial infarction" when the appropriate clinical picture is present. If diagnostic criteria are clear and comprehensive, then a diagnosis can be made with certainty when they are met in an individual patient. Problems arise when diagnostic criteria are not clear, when the doctor is not sure what they are, or when there is difficulty in eliciting the relevant symptoms, signs and abnormal laboratory results. But there is a sense in which Popper's views are applicable in this field. For even when we have created a diagnostic class, and given it a name, it is as well to recognize its potential incompleteness, and to look for sub-classes within it (e.g., AIDS patients with or without the virus) as their recognition may further aid the management of patients if either the response to treatment, possibility of prevention, or the prognosis is different in the different sub-classes.

I question two other points made by Lanes. First, it is not true that knowledge advances only by showing that a theory is false, although many great advances have been made in this way. It also advances when sound hypotheses, that is, those that appear to be the best solutions to particular problems, are tested rigorously and withstand repeated attempts at their falsification. There are many current theories that have not been shown to be false, and that may indeed be true. Their formulation and testing have constituted an advance in our knowledge and understanding. I reject Stove's statement[1] that the word "knowledge" only applies to something known to be true; we can have knowledge of current hypotheses and of the data on which these hypotheses are based. Second, Lanes' use of the term "corroboration" to imply confirmation, as in his discussion of the bacillus-melanoma theory, is not the sense in which Popper intended the word to be used.[7] For Popper the degree of corroboration of a theory corresponds to the extent to which the theory has resisted rigorous attempts to falsify it, rather than mere repetition of the same basic observation. Corroboration, even in Popper's sense, does not confirm a theory or increase the probability that a theory is true, but it does strengthen the theory and will increase our preference for it over other theories that have not withstood such critical examination.

Falsification, Verification and Causal Inference in Epidemiology

My problems with Susser's paper began with the statement:

Popper argues that science advances by the process of deduction alone. We begin with a hypothesis—an act of invention and imagination—and can reach a conclusion only to the extent that the hypothesis can be rejected.

The first sentence is clearly erroneous, as Popper has repeatedly argued that science advances by conjecture and refutation—

by the proposal of hypotheses and by rigorous attempts to falsify them. Furthermore, while hypotheses may be acts of invention and imagination they may also be the results of reasoned argument and critical review of available information; and while conclusions as to their *truth* may be reached only by refutation, conclusions about the value of a hypothesis as a basis for action can be made on the basis of its ability to withstand critical attempts at falsification. Corroboration in this sense increases our preference for the hypothesis. Surely logic dictates that failure to falsify does not affirm a theory. Failure to find a black swan does not mean that none exists; indeed, black swans do exist in Australia.

What are we to make of the two important aspects in which Susser differs from Popper's position—the asymmetry between falsification and corroboration, and the matter of induction. I do not understand the statement "the high risk procedure of disproof by deduction is not less fallible than that of verification or proof." You cannot *disprove* scientific statements by deduction but only by testing them, although you may know that they have already been refuted as the result of previous experiments. Furthermore, you cannot verify or *prove* hypotheses by testing them; you can only demonstrate that your tests do not refute them. While Susser may be able to remember experimental results that have been incompatible with the truth of a given hypothesis, can he quote any which could be said to have verified or to have *proved* the hypothesis under consideration? I suspect not; instead the results would have been considered to have strengthened the hypothesis, even to the extent that important actions might be taken.

Preference is not established by the process of induction—indeed I was startled by the suggestion that "every probability statement about a sample population must be extrapolated by induction to become a general statement." Before any measurements are made on a sample population we must choose which measurements will be made; this process suggests a hypothetico-deductive rather than an inductive approach. Indeed, the measurements are often chosen to test a particular hypothesis, and the results will therefore tend to refute or to corroborate the hypothesis, the degree of corroboration depending on the rigor with which the hypothesis is tested. When measurements are made that are not intended as tests of the hypothesis, statements about the results are difficult to justify, even as statements of probability. The results of such measurements do provide a legitimate basis for the formulation of a new hypothesis. They do not, however, demand extrapolation by induction into a general statement, and I believe that most epidemiologists would reject this suggestion.

In his discussion of probability Susser states that "a hypothesis must be clearly formulated before testing, and the aim is to reject the null hypothesis of no difference." Rejection of the null hypothesis is chosen for ease and convenience, as other types of hypothesis tend to be more difficult to test. It is true that studies in which conventionally set limits of statistical significance are not met are likely to be given short shrift. But it is also obvious, on logical as well as traditional statistical grounds, that achievement of "statistical significance" does not constitute proof or verification. Neither does failure to achieve it mean that the hypothesis is incorrect. Methodologic problems may affect the results in either direction, and when statistical significance is reached it may be for reasons that have nothing to do with the original hypothesis. Several of these points are made by Susser himself, but he still considers that a statistically significant result "affirms" the hypothesis. Perhaps we use the word "affirm" in different ways.

When dealing with "Strength of Association" Susser argues that "the stronger the relation, the less a confounding variable capable of explaining the association is likely to exist." Unfortunately no matter how strong the relation appears, we cannot conclude that such a variable doesn't exist. For this reason the strength of the relation cannot affirm the hypothesis, although it may make it preferable to other hypotheses. We may do many experiments at sea level that appear to "affirm" the statement that "pure water boils at 100° C." Clearly they do not affirm that particular statement because if we were to change atmospheric pressure we would get a different result. We could, of course, change the hypothesis, but the new one also could not be affirmed, although we might be getting closer to the truth. A similar argument can be made for the relation of cola-coloring in babies to maternal exposure to PCB. The resulting hypothesis that PCB is the cause of cola-coloring may be true, but we cannot be sure that there was not a contaminating chemical. In practice this apparent indeterminacy is of little consequence. If the hypothesis has withstood rigorous testing then it would be sensible to try and prevent maternal exposure to PCB. Popper does not argue that "affirmative results in the same direction indicate no more than survival of the hypothesis." He would not use the adjective "affirmative" for the reasons presented above, but he would accept corroboration (in the sense of survival following rigorous testing) as a basis for preferring the hypothesis and for acting on it if necessary.

Most of Susser's paper seems to be an argument in favor of the "affirmation" or "verification" of theories. He argues that this is what epidemiologists do, and that it is what they ought to do. He finishes by stating "the formalities of philosophy need to be tempered by good epidemiologic sense." But are his views good sense, and does it really matter in practice whether one is concerned about affirmation and verification, rather than falsification, refutation and corroboration? I think it does. The problem with the idea of verification is that it implies that we know the truth about something even if it is conceded that we do not know the whole truth about it. When we believe that our knowledge is secure it is difficult not to become a little complacent and dogmatism tends to replace doubt. In scientific research belief in our ideas may cause us to search for observations that support them, and to avoid crucial tests which may destroy them. Many authors of scientific papers ignore work that appears to contradict their own views. This is not just bad science but a form of intellectual dishonesty. I believe it stems from a fear of refutation and of the exposure of error. Verification and affirmation are approaches that make the path easier—unfortunately so, if it leads in the wrong direction!

In clinical practice reliance on theory, and belief in ideas, have led us to persist with many remedies that we now consider useless. These remedies have been used because doctors have *be-*

lieved in them. Surely we would do better if our main concern was the search for error, in clinical practice as well as in research; this concept has been for me the main message of Popper's writings.[8] For this and other reasons I do not believe that "verification" is the right approach for epidemiologists or for other scientists. Rational argument based on a continual and constant search for errors should be the basis of epidemiologic research. Popper has pointed us in the right direction if that is the path we wish to follow.

References

1. Stove DC. Karl Popper and the Jazz Age. Encounter, 1985 June:65–74.

2. Popper KR. *The Logic of Scientific Discovery*. Revised ed. New York: Harper & Row, 1968. Originally published as *Logik der Forschung*. Vienna: Springer, 1934.

3. Popper KR. *Objective Knowledge: an Evolutionary Approach*. Oxford: Clarendon Press, 1972.

4. Popper KR. *Conjectures and Refutations: the Growth of Scientific Knowledge*. New York: Harper Torchbooks, 1963.

5. Schilpp PA., ed. *The Philosophy of Karl Popper, Vol. 2*. La Salle, Il: Open Court, 1974:1025.

6. Magee B. *Popper*. London: Fontana/Collins, 1973.

7. Popper KR. *Realism and the Aim of Science*. London: Hutchinson, 1983:243.

8. McIntyre N. Popper KR. The critical attitude in medicine: the need for a new ethics. Br Med J 1983;287:1919–1923.

The Implications of Alternative Views About Causal Inference for the Work of the Practicing Epidemiologist

Diana B. Petitti

Division of Family and Community Medicine
University of California at San Francisco
School of Medicine
San Francisco, California

Mostly I am either bored or confused by discussions of philosophy, and no less by discussions of the philosophy of science than by discussions of whether particulars or eternal universals are transient and insubstantial.[1] My initial response to the papers in this volume was "Who cares?" On re-reading the papers after a summer spent doing non-epidemiological work, I have a different view. If it is conceded that a major goal of epidemiology is to understand cause, then the discussions in this volume show that a choice between the Popperian (refutationist) and the inductive (verificationist) approach to epidemiology has profound implications for the way in which the practicing epidemiologist carries out his or her day-to-day work. Before illustrating with some examples, I should explain why I worked this summer at some tasks other than epidemiology.

Like many epidemiologists, I spend a high percentage of my time reviewing manuscripts reporting the results of studies done by others, reviewing proposals for new studies, sitting on advisory committees to decide what actions ought to be taken based on the results of epidemiologic studies, and helping others deal with data from their own epidemiologic studies. In all of these activities, I have found less and less evidence of scientific creativity and more and more striking deficits in the understanding of biology and the other sciences that relate closely to epidemiology. The literature of epidemiology increasingly is becoming an archive of the results of information derived from mechanical applications of multivariate analysis. Studies are proposed solely to "fill holes" in the literature, tabulating every exposure against every disease. Actions are based on an appraisal of epidemiologic studies according to checklists based entirely on the technical aspects of the studies. Investigators are more interested in the mechanics of data analysis than in the substance of the issues being addressed.

This spring, these impressions led me to view epidemiology as a field that is in trouble as a scientific discipline and one from which I needed a rest. I perceive now with a clarity I lacked upon my first reading of the papers in this volume, and before my summer spent at a distance from the pressures of participation in the field, that the practical application of what can be learned from these philosophical discussions may help to remedy some of the problems with the evolution of epidemiology over the past few years. Specifically, I believe that fixing firmly in mind the refutationist philosophy formulated by Popper and using it to guide the choice of what to do as an epidemiologist might salvage epidemiology from demise.

The difference between what I shall call the Popperian practice of epidemiology and the inductivist practice of epidemiology can be illustrated with a hypothetical example of a graduate student seeking a topic for a thesis project. She is interested in studying breast cancer, probably because an aunt died of it, but she has no specific project in mind. A Popperian student, that is, one who attempts to conduct science by actively employing the process of conjecture and refutation, reads about the epidemiology, endocrinology, molecular biology, sociology, and psychology of breast cancer. Based on this reading, she formulates a testable hypothesis about breast cancer, and she then collects data that would, using Popper's language, corroborate or refute this hypothesis. An inductivist student, that is, one who believes that scientific theories become established through the gradual accretion of data verifying the theory, reviews only the literature on the epidemiology of breast cancer. She need not formulate testable hypothesis to conduct her research, but merely needs to collect more data on breast cancer in relation to possible risk factors, either replicating previous findings or finding some as yet unexamined variables to analyze. Knowledge gained from the study is, for the Popperian student, tentative and theoretical, and the data serve only to refute the tentative gropings toward this theoretical knowledge. For the inductivist student, the knowledge resides in the cumulating data, and more data means more knowledge. The questionnaires that a Popperian epidemiologist uses in his or her studies can be short, because each question is directed to a specific hypothesis. A Popperian study, having specifically targeted scientific objectives, can be less expensive than that of an inductivist, because the amount of data that is collected based on prespecified hypotheses is less than that based on a desire to relate everything to anything.

The crucial distinction is the difference between scientific knowledge and factual knowledge: Science is better described as a system of abstract theories than as an agglomeration of factual observations. The results of an analysis of the relationship of 20 variables with the risk of acute myocardial infarction should not be considered a contribution to the advancement of science just because the relationship of these variables with myocardial infarction is previously unknown. An epidemiologist should not seek funds for a study of the relationship of Asian ethnicity with the risk of prostate cancer based simply on the argument that "we know that the risk of prostatic cancer is higher in Blacks than in Whites, but we don't know the risk in Asians."

In taking the Popperian viewpoint, many of the things that could be done using epidemiologic methods are things that would not be done; accumulation of data without the formulation of testable theories about disease causation would seldom be worthwhile from this philosophical base. The consequences may be fewer publications, fewer consultations, and more library work, but the consequences may also be more productive research and more rapid advances in the accumulation of scientific knowledge.[2]

References

1. Schlesinger GN. Scientists and philosophy. In this volume.

2. Platt JR. Strong inference. Science 1964;146:348–353.

Induction Does Not Exist in Epidemiology, Either

Charles Poole

Epidemiology Resources Inc.
Chestnut Hill, Massachusetts

George Schlesinger, the only full-time philosopher among this monograph's four principal essayists, offers the paradoxically practical advice that scientists should not expect practical advice from philosophers of science.[1] Several epidemiologic counterexamples falsify this claim. "Causal inference" is an inherently philosophical activity about which epidemiologists have a decidedly pragmatic attitude. We want to know if checklists of causal criteria "work," in the sense of bringing us closer to the truth about epidemiologic theories. We sometimes ask whether it is useful to measure our personal feelings of certainty and doubt about these theories. These and other issues in causal inference are matters for both pragmatic and philosophical consideration.

I am against the use of causal criteria and Bayesian analysis in epidemiology. I do not think that any characteristic of an exposure-disease association can make it objectively more or less likely to be causal. I find the argument compelling that we cannot increase our knowledge of the causes of disease by quantifying our feelings. I think that the best way of interpreting epidemiologic research for scientific and policy purposes is to engage in rational, critical discussion of causal theories.

The case for critical discussion in epidemiology begins with

Popper's argument that induction is a myth. The nonexistence of induction has dire implications for the empirical "affirmation" of theories and for subjective "methods" of quantitative introspection. Elsewhere in this monograph, Lanes summarizes Popper's arguments against induction and illustrates them with epidemiologic examples.[2] My tack is to offer a direct criticism of the affirmative case for induction that has been put forth by its epidemiologic advocates.

Popper claims to have learned from Hume that induction does not exist. Some epidemiologists, siding with Bacon, counter that inductive reasoning is quite useful in epidemiology. This rejoinder misses the mark. If Popper had claimed that mermaids do not exist, it would not refute his claim to reply that these creatures are quite useful to drowning sailors. We may grant the utility of mermaids in principle without conceding their existence. To refute the claim that mermaids are imaginary, we need to show a mermaid; we can worry about her usefulness later.

Is there an epidemiologic counterexample with which to refute Popper's assertion that induction is a fairy tale? In his contribution to the monograph, Susser claims to have found two: probability statements and the generation of causal hypotheses.[3]

Probability Statements

Susser reiterates Jacobsen's claim that probability statements are examples of inductive reasoning in epidemiology.[4] Both authors refer to the frequency or sampling interpretation of probability that is manifest in the p-values and confidence limits with which all epidemiologists are familiar. The argument seems to be that we compute and interpret p-values and confidence limits because we want to draw inferences from samples (the particular) to populations (the general). I do not deny the existence of this desire. I simply wish to point out that p-values and confidence limits do not satisfy it.

According to Cox and Hinkley, statistical analysis begins with the selection of a family of probability models.[5] The selection of this family is not a trivial task; but once the selection has been made, it is to be "assumed provisionally that the data are indeed derived from one of the models" in the chosen family. The assumed family member provides a set of theoretical expectations for our observations. The p-values and confidence limits we compute are merely deduced from the models that we have taken, so to speak, off the shelf.[6]

Consider for example a series of four flips of a coin. Of the many theories that could provide expectations for the outcome of this series, consider just these two:

A. The coin has a head on each side.

B. The coin is balanced, it has a head on one side and a tail on the other, and it is flipped fairly.

Now consider the five possible outcomes of the series of four flips, disregarding the order of the flips:

1. No heads

2. One head

3. Two heads

4. Three heads

5. Four heads

Theory A predicts that outcome 5 will occur with a probability of one and assigns a uniform probability of zero to outcomes 1 through 4. Theory B conforms to a member of the family of binomial models that predicts a probability of 0.0625 for outcomes 1 and 5, a probability of 0.25 for outcomes 2 and 4, and a probability of 0.375 for outcome 3.

Now suppose we flip the coin four times and observe four heads (outcome 5). The p-value corresponding to this observation under theory A is 1.0. Can we conclude that theory A is true? I think not.

A more conventional analysis would focus on theory B. Can we conclude from our observation of outcome 5 that the probability is 0.0625 that theory B is true? A first-year statistics student might be tempted to do so, but would quickly learn otherwise.

The statement, "p = 0.0625," is a deduction from theory B. It tells us something about a real or hypothetical population of series of four coin flips only under the provisional assumption that theory B is indeed true. No p-value or confidence limit can tell us anything more. No probability statement, inside or outside of epidemiology, is an inductive generalization from a sample to a population.

The idea that statements of sampling probability are inductive is reflected in the common misinterpretation of the null p-value as the probability that the null hypothesis is true. This interpretation is incorrect because the null p-value is computed under the assumption that the null hypothesis *is* true. Confidence limits are linked to hypotheses other than the null by identically deductive reasoning.

Hypothesis Generation

Susser's second nomination reiterates Davies' claim that "forming hypotheses based on observation" is an important example of inductive reasoning in epidemiology.[7] This notion is quite popular. It is embodied in such expressions as "hypothesis-generating study" and the supposedly important distinction between hypotheses that are "suggested by the data" and those that are suggested in some other way.

The basic idea is that we compute exposure-disease associations in data sets and look at them. Some of the associations suggest causal theories to us. The suggestion may be made by a measure of association that does not equal its null value (e.g., an incidence rate ratio that does not equal one) or by a p-value that is less than a value that has been determined in advance to confer statistical significance to an association.

The purportedly distinctive characteristic of this method of generating hypotheses is that it "starts from" the data and "goes to" the hypothesis. Because it is the observed association that is doing the talking (metaphorically at least), the epidemiologist has only to be a good listener. The ability to hear the hypotheses that data suggest becomes manifest as creativity and imagination. It is neither required nor even desirable for a hypothesis to be in the listener's mind before the data speak.

Theory-free observation, in fact, is the hallmark of this version of "reasoning from the particular to the general." Induction needs this property to set itself apart from "retroduction," which is a way of generating hypotheses that relies on deductions from earlier hypotheses.[8]

Retroduction goes like this: We start with a set of theories, even in the form of vaguely formulated expectations. We then make epidemiologic observations in the form of one or more exposure-disease associations. We see that some of these observations clash with our expectations. It is here that creativity and imagination enter, not as an ability to listen to data but as an ability to solve a problem. To solve the problem of the inconsistency between theory and observation, we invent a new theory.

Popper is sometimes accused of neglecting the question of the origin of theories, but he actually has much to say about it. His answer is that theories come from the minds of human beings and not from data. Popper denies the occurrence of any theory-free observation that would be required for the psychological process of induction to work. He claims that "[a]n observation always presupposes the existence of some system of expectations"[9] and that "there is no such thing as an unprejudiced observation . . . no such thing as passive experience . . . no such thing as a perception except in the context of interests and expectations, and hence of regularities or 'laws'".[10] All observations are theory-laden, our earliest and most primitive theories being inborn expectations such as those that babies and animals exhibit.

Ironically, induction's defenders sometimes give the same argument that leads Popper to deny its existence. Consider the following statement by Hanson:

Natural scientists do not 'start from' hypotheses. They start from data. And not even from ordinary commonplace data—but from surprising anomalies. Thus Aristotle remarks that knowledge begins in astonishment. Peirce makes perplexity the trigger of scientific inquiry. And James and Dewey treat intelligence as the result of mastering problem situations.[11]

Hanson appears at first to be defending induction, but as he continues he provides the same argument that Popper uses to attack it. How can an observation be surprising, anomalous, astonishing, perplexing, or problematic unless it contradicts some expectation? And what could this prior expectation be but a prediction from an existing theory, however humbly expressed or incompletely realized at the time of the observation?

Every epidemiologic hypothesis that appears to arise inductively "from the data" actually arises from a clash between the data and an existing theoretical expectation. When MacMahon et al.[12] saw an association between coffee drinking and cancer of the pancreas in their data, they were surprised because it contradicted their theoretical expectation that coffee should *not* be associated with this disease.

It was MacMahon et al., not their data, who suggested the alternative causal hypothesis. They reasoned not from the particular observation in their study to the general causal conjecture, but from their prior *noncausal* conjecture to an expectation of *nonassociation*. This expectation was not fulfilled in their data, so they responded with another theory in the form of a causal hypothesis. They practiced retroduction, not induction.

It sometimes takes very little to generate a theory. In fact, the feat can be accomplished without any data at all. For example, I shall now generate a causal theory: "Thalidomide causes angiosarcoma of the liver." (As though it mattered, I hereby stipulate that I have never seen any data relating angiosarcoma of the liver to thalidomide.) Some theories require great imagination to be generated. Others require almost none, but once stated they are "generated" nevertheless. Hypotheses formed by filling in the blanks in the statement, "Exposure E causes disease D," fall into the latter category.

As Hanson emphasized,[11] I need offer no reason for *accepting* my theory about thalidomide and angiosarcoma of the liver to justify my *suggesting* it. There may be a popular notion that to suggest a theory is to express a personal commitment to it. If this notion were true, we might never see an epidemiologic study funded or conducted by industry. When we ask what kind of evidence is necessary for a certain hypothesis to be considered generated, we are really asking what kind of evidence is necessary for a hypothesis that has already been generated to be considered seriously. We should not confuse considering a hypothesis seriously with generating a hypothesis.

Section 5 of the Toxic Substances Control Act[13] stipulates a large class of causal theories for which there can be no prior observation. These theories concern possible health effects of chemicals that have not yet been synthesized. The concern that motivates the generation of theories about health effects of chemicals that do not yet exist is reasonable, even though there would seem to be no reason to accept any one of these theories until we are told at least the chemical structure of the compound in question. (The Administrator of the Environmental Protection Agency gets 90 days to decide whether any such theory should be tested empirically before the new chemical goes onto the market.)

In even the most highly mechanized and seemingly hypothesis-free "fishing expedition" in epidemiology, the hypotheses are suggested before the correlation coefficients, relative risks, or p-values are ever computed. The hypotheses are generated by the mere selection of the diseases and exposures to evaluate.

Consider for instance the "hypothesis-generating study" by Siemiatycki et al. of nineteen varieties of cancer and nine kinds of organic dusts.[14] These diseases and exposures were selected for reasons; the reasons combine to "suggest" 171 causal and 171 preventive hypotheses. The investigators describe their task as "to determine whether there seem to be any remarkable cancer-exposure associations." That they separate the remarkable from the unremarkable belies any description of their work as free of prior hypotheses. At one point the authors state, "Whether a given piece of evidence comes from an hypothesis-generating or an hypothesis-testing study *per se* is irrelevant."

My conjecture is that a study is called a hypothesis-generating study whenever the investigators have formed the judgment that the evidence produced by the study does not constitute a strong test of any hypothesis. "Hypothesis-generating" has become a code for "weakly hypothesis-testing." There is a similar connotation to the occasional warning that certain data are to be "interpreted with caution." A literal reading of such language, of course, would imply that all other data are to interpreted with reckless abandon.

Developers of statistical methods of exploratory data analysis (EDA), an effort to systematize the derivation of hypotheses from data, also reveal the existence of the expectations that accompany every examination of data. Leamer's "model of inference" for "specification searching" begins with "preconscious innate propositions."[15] Diaconis urges the adoption of "working hypotheses" in EDA.[16] Good's philosophy of EDA presupposes a distinction between patterns in data that are "mere coincidences" and patterns for which other hypotheses should be developed.[17] Like any other analyst of data, the practitioner of EDA goes into the analysis with the expectation of separating one kind of pattern from another. The existence of such expectations means that retroduction, not induction, is being practiced.

Conclusion

Neither the frequency interpretation of probability statements nor the generation of causal hypotheses stands up as an example of induction in epidemiology. P-values and confidence limits are deduced from probability models. Hypotheses are suggested by people, not by data. Data play a role in the suggestion of hypotheses by failing to conform to existing theoretical expectations and thereby creating problems for other theories to solve. Popper's claim of the nonexistence of induction remains unrefuted by epidemiologic counterexamples.

It has been the purpose of this essay to ask whether p-values and hypothesis generation are inductive, not to pass judgment on their merit. To describe statements of sampling probability as deductive and epidemiologic hypotheses as retroductive is neither to support nor to deny the utility of either aspect of epidemiologic practice. (It is useful to be pushed to shore after a shipwreck, whether it is a mermaid or a dolphin that does the pushing.) On the other hand, we should be skeptical of Susser and Schlesinger's implicit claim that if scientists are doing something it must be the preferable thing to do. There are alternatives to sampling probabilities and "hypothesis-generating" studies.

The subjective interpretation of probability is an alternative to the sampling interpretation. Strong tests of smaller numbers of hypotheses are an alternative to weak tests of larger numbers. Such questions are beyond the scope of this essay, as are the larger issues of causal criteria and subjectivity in epidemiology, to which I alluded in the introduction. One of my reasons for choosing such a narrow topic as the two ostensible examples of induction is to provide a contrast with the overly extensive treatment of philosophical issues we are accustomed to seeing in epidemiology. Almost without exception, papers on causal inference have attempted to cover the entire subject. The result has been great breadth and precious little depth.

After Jacobsen and Davies asserted that p-values and hypothesis generation are inductive, Maclure denied their claims.[18] He did so briefly, however, as his goal also was to present a comprehensive overview. In the present monograph, Susser devotes no more than a paragraph to reiterating Jacobsen's and Davies' claims. He does not mention Maclure's counter assertions.

I harbor no delusion that this essay will be the last word on induction in epidemiology. I do suggest, however, that if philosophy can nourish epidemiologic practice, it will do so in pieces that are small enough for us to chew.

References

1. Schlesinger G. Scientists and philosophy. In this volume.

2. Lanes SF. The logic of causal inference in medicine. In this volume.

3. Susser M. Falsification, verification and causal inference in epidemiology: reconsiderations in the light of Sir Karl Popper's philosophy. In this volume.

4. Jacobsen M. Against Popperized epidemiology. Int J Epidemiol 1975;4:159–168.

5. Cox DR, Hinkley DV. *Theoretical Statistics*. London: Chapman and Hall, 1974.

6. Fisher RA. The logic of inductive inference (with discussion). J R Stat Soc 1935;98:39–82.

7. Davies AM. Comments on "Popper's philosophy for epidemiologists." Comment one. Int J Epidemiol 1975;4:169–170.

8. Peirce C. In: Hawthorne C, et al., eds. *Collected Works*. Vol. II, Bk. III, Ch. 2, Pt. 3. Cambridge, MA: Harvard University Press, 1931–58.

9. Popper KR. *Objective Knowledge: An Evolutionary Approach.* Oxford: Clarendon Press, 1983:344.

10. Popper K. *Unended Quest: An Intellectual Autobiography.* La Salle, Illinois: Open Court, 1976:51–52.

11. Hanson NR. The logic of discovery. J Phil 1958;55:1073–1089.

12. MacMahon B, Yen S, Trichopoulos D, et al. Coffee and cancer of the pancreas. N Engl J Med 1981;304:630–633.

13. Public Law 94-469, 90 Statute 2003, 15 United States Code Section 2601 (1976).

14. Siemiatycki J, Richardson L, Gerin M, et al. Associations between several sites of cancer and nine organic dusts: results from an hypothesis-generating case-control study in Montreal, 1979–1983. Am J Epidemiol 1986;123:235–249.

15. Leamer EE. *Specification Searches: Ad Hoc Inference With Nonexperimental Data.* New York: John Wiley & Sons, 1978:16–20.

16. Diaconis P. Theories of data analysis: from magical thinking through classical statistics. Chapter 1 in: Hoaglin DC, Mosteller F, Tukey JW, eds. *Exploring Data Tables, Trends and Shapes.* New York: John Wiley & Sons, Inc., 1985.

17. Good IJ. The philosophy of exploratory data analysis. Phil Sci 1983;50:283–295.

18. Maclure M. Popperian refutation in epidemiology. Am J Epidemiol 1985;121:343–350.

REJOINDER

There's a Fascination Frantic in Philosophical Fancies

George N. Schlesinger

Department of Philosophy
University of North Carolina
Chapel Hill, North Carolina

James Boswell relates that when presented with "Bishop Berkeley's ingenious sophistry to prove the non-existence of matter . . . Johnson answered, striking his foot with mighty force against a large stone, till he rebounded from it, 'I refute him *thus*.'" For over 200 years, commentators have been grappling with the task of articulating the ideas that lay beneath this famous performance by England's greatest man of letters. I submit that, among other things, Dr. Johnson may have wished to indicate how much he preferred a sore foot over the agony of an attempt at philosophical rebuttal.

On another occasion, upon learning about the second marriage of an acquaintance, the witty sage quipped that it was "the triumph of hope over experience." The same might well be said about this Rejoinder, written in the wake of the chastening experience of seeing the points I have tried to make tenaciously disregarded by some of the eminent discussants.

I shall try to refrain from making any pronouncement on what epidemiologists should do, or ought to believe. I shall, however, state that as a matter of experience I have found that many outstanding workers in the health related disciplines, as well as in the empirical sciences in general, have been interested not only in producing the maximum amount of publishable results but also in gaining some measure of insight into the logical structure, covert presuppositions and the metaphysical foundations of their discipline. They, unlike several of the distinguished discussants in this volume, have realized that philosophy was supposed to be devoted to purely conceptual analysis and had not expected philosophers to provide them with handy tips about the best research methods to adopt. (A preeminent medical scientist who has seen the penultimate version of this Note expressed his concern as to whether my statement that philosophy is devoted to purely conceptual analysis is going to be much of a help. "In the minds of the epidemiologists 'conceptual analysis' may include everything they do" he commented. Unfortunately there is no neat solution to this problem. The most I feel able to add is the suggestion that "conceptual analysis" is the name commonly assigned to the painstaking, clarificationary process of abstract obscurities. Conceptual analysis might be said to constitute a pure armchair activity; it is supposed to be a rigorous endeavour to unsnarl ideational tangles.) Regarding themselves to be reflective creatures, who do not live by bread alone, they simply succumbed to the temptation of having the intellectual satisfaction deriving from a dispassionate inquiry into the ultimate justification of their methodology, and into the rational grounds for their claims, and wish to partake in the kind of fulfillment likely to result from a deeper understanding of the validation and of the significance of their work.

Perhaps we should remind ourselves that most of the great, creative scientists did not regard practicality to be the main purpose even of the empirical sciences. Henri Poincaré, for instance, said:

The scientist does not study nature because it is useful to do so. He studies it because he takes pleasure in it; and he takes pleasure in it because it is beautiful. If nature were not beautiful, it would not be worth knowing and life would not be worth living.[1]

Professor Maclure has pointed out that my ". . . view is refuted by well-documented examples." Thus it should certainly be futile for me to attempt arguing against solid facts. He goes even further and claims that my view is also refuted by *myself*. In the beginning of my paper I have maintained that a scientist cannot expect to improve his experimental techniques and problem-solving skills through the study of philosophy, yet later I concede that philosophy may have a profound impact on a scientist's attitudes. Is this not an outright contradiction? No, and I am afraid it may appear so only to someone who has meticulously missed the entire point of the paper.

Let me try to explain. Not too many of our Congressmen or Senators have much time or inclination to read poetry and even those who do would not be able to see that it had a bearing on their law-making activities. Yet one of the most often quoted sayings of Shelley has been "Poets are the unacknowledged legislators of the world." What does it mean? Shelley is not suggesting that our solons do, or ought to, consult their poetry books before deciding what laws to vote for. What he does imply is that in a rather *indirect* manner the works of poets have an effect on the deliberations of politicians. The cultural climate we live in, the way we feel about things, is partially influenced by the impact poetry makes upon the human mind. Poetry is a significant factor in shaping our fundamental assumptions about right and wrong, and these in turn play a role in determining the laws of the land. It seems to me that T.S. Eliot's saying ". . . morals are open to being altered by literature"[2] should be interpreted in a similar fashion.

Philosophy may be said to play a parallel regulative role. For example, throughout the Middle Ages relatively little progress was made in the natural sciences. Surely this stasis cannot be attributed to the fact that for over a thousand years there existed no gifted individuals comparable to the great scientists of the last 300 years. What stood in the way of the rapid development of physics, chemistry and so on, was mainly the metaphysical presuppositions generally held in those days concerning the proper use to be made of one's intellectual capacities and the limits of human reason and understanding. It was widely held that there was little to be known beyond what was already known to the great minds of classical antiquity. Thus, not much was discovered, since not much was attempted to be discovered. This example illustrates the immense power philosophy may sometimes have in shaping our ends. But to improve a scientist's experimental techniques or problem solving skills? Most unlikely!

We should perhaps concentrate on the most profound misunderstandings displayed by several discussants, namely, those relating to the nature and status of induction. It is unfortunate that it should cause sorrow and even anger to some leading medical scientists, e.g., Professors Maclure and McIntyre, but we have to face the fact that it is not merely ludicrously wrong to maintain that induction is a myth; it is rather that the scientist does not ever take a single step without relying on induction. Indeed, his unbridled commitment to the principle that the future will be like the past, that is, the principle of the uniformity of nature or briefly the principle of induction, is so all embracing that even when he wishes sometimes to falsify a hypothesis he does so on the basis of his firm conviction of the validity of that principle.

To keep matters as simple as possible let us presuppose only the most general definition of the principle of induction, which as everybody knows is to assume that the unobserved will be like the observed, or that the future will be like the past, or even that like things are alike. Also let me refer to a very simple hypothesis that all would agree has been most intensely falsified, namely Aristotle's hypothesis according to which the heavier a terrestrial body the greater its downward acceleration. How, one might ask, has the hypothesis been refuted? First by Galileo, and subsequently through thousands of experiments performed with different objects in different locations showing that in fact whatever the weight of an object, its acceleration near the surface of the earth equals g. Suppose now that someone asks: surely all these experiments have taken place in the *past*, how then can one say to have shown Aristotle's hypothesis not to be true *at all*? The principle, that heavier bodies fall faster than lighter bodies, could still very well be obeyed tomorrow, next week, or in fact at all times in the future? The obvious answer is that we assume by the rule of induction that the future will be like the past, and if Aristotle's law did not hold in the past, it will not hold in the future either.

Clearly, therefore, a scientist could never believe to have falsified any theory unless he made the *entirely unprovable* assumption that whatever has been observed to be false here and now is false everywhere, at all times; that the world can be relied upon not to change from place to place, and from the past and present to the future, i.e., that the laws of nature remain constant throughout space and time.

Here it is relevant to mention that I have found Maclure's claim to have discovered yet another contradiction in my paper simply mind-boggling. He cites no less than four passages in my article where I explicitly refer to the act of refutation in philosophy and mathematics as decisive, and this blatantly clashes with my attempts to detract from its all-absorbing paramountcy in epidemiology. A brief reply to this, clearly, should include mention of the fact that in philosophy or in mathematics refutation does not require presupposing the uniformity of nature, the principle of homogeneity, or (to use J.R. Lucas's recent expression[3]) the principle of the causal inefficacy of space and time, or the assumption that the physical world will behave in the future and in distant places similar to the way it does here and now. In other words, while the empirical sciences are totally dependent on inductive logic, the logic of analytic philosophy and of mathematics is deductive.

Those remaining few who are still bent upon defending some version of the grandiose claim that induction is a myth have sometimes attempted advocating the more modest thesis that as a matter of wise *strategy*, it is always preferable to try to falsify a hypothesis than to confirm it. Thus their contention has been that while logically neither confirmation nor falsification is justified, the practical scientist, who does not aspire to deductive rigor, will succeed faster if he invariably seeks to refute, rather than confirm, putative theories.

There are only two things wrong with the revised thesis. First, even if it was correct, it would amount to something like a useful trick of the trade, without much particular philosophical interest. Secondly, it is incorrect. The following may serve as useful illustrative examples:

1) Kepler came to hold the profound conviction that the different amounts of time it took the various planets to complete their orbit around the sun was not of a random value; he assumed these periods to be determined by some law, even though he had no idea by what law. He did *not* set out to refute his conjecture—indeed it is hard to see how he might have gone about doing such a thing. On the contrary, he kept for many years assiduously trying to *verify* his hunch. At long last he hit upon the idea that the squares of revolution-periods are functions of the cubes of the mean distances of the planets from the sun. The hypothesis, known as Kepler's third law, is regarded until this very day to be true, and no reasonable scientist is planning any experiments to refute it.

2) One of the greatest ideas introduced into physics in the 19th century was that of lines and fields of force. Faraday believed that there can be no such thing as action at a distance. He had the intuition that a body acts on its immediate neighbor, which again acts on the point next to it, and so on. Faraday had no evidence for his thesis concerning the transmission of magnetic and electrical forces. Subsequently, Maxwell was greatly impressed by Faraday's suggestion, so much so that he, rather than trying to falsify it, tried for 20 years to formulate it mathematically and to confirm it. He ended up with the epoch-making Maxwell's equation on the basis of which he was able to predict that electricity and magnetism can propagate waves. Those predictions turned out eventually to be true and have at last provided the empirical *vindication* of Faraday's *conjecture.*

3) Among the indefinitely many examples from the present century, let me refer briefly to H. Weyl's suggestion of a geometrical invariance for the electromagnetic potential $A\mu$. The particular formulation of this theory was blatantly contradicted by experimental evidence. Did this apparent refutation lead to the rejection of his conjecture? No, many physicists found it to be too beautiful to be wrong. They agreed with Dirac's famous dictum "It is more important to have beauty in one's equation than to

have them fit the experiments." After the invention of quantum mechanics it became indeed evident that Weyl's instincts were basically on target, and the correct expression was produced for his scale factor.

4) As we move in the direction of epidemiology, we might remind ourselves of the work of the great Paul Ehrlich. Ehrlich held the firm conviction that there must be certain substances that could function as "magic bullets," destroying particular, dangerous bacteria, while doing no harm to the patient's body. Decades of hard work by thousands of scientists failed to achieve what Ehrlich saw as the objective of all medical art. The many setbacks, however, sowed no doubts in his mind that his aim would be achieved and he was even quite certain about the way one had to go about achieving it. Millions of people owe Ehrlich a debt of gratitude for not having adopted a falsificationist scientific methodology!

I sincerely hope that Drs. Labarthe and Stallones, who say "Schlesinger appears to enjoy, and perhaps welcome the devastation [of Popper]," are prepared to believe me that I have not been harboring any sentiments of *schadenfreude* in the remotest sense of that word. I do not even remember having read a single word of Popper in the last 15 years or so, and am not absolutely certain that he has said all the ludicrous things associated with his name. But are we then to understand that the devout Popperians who have contributed to this volume have also misrepresented their mentor? To pick but one of a very large number of examples, Dr. Lanes, for instance, states on the first page of his paper:

> In recognizing scientific knowledge as conjecture that can be seen as false, but never as true or probable, Popper explains the uncertainty inherent in all our knowledge. . . .

I assume that the basic laws of logic are not being claimed to have been overthrown. Thus let us suppose that statements p and q are contradictories (i.e., $\sim p \leftrightarrow q$, or that p is false if and only if q is true). Suppose also that scientist Alvarez advances the conjecture that p, while another physicist, Basov, stren-

uously denies it, insisting that on the contrary, it is the conjecture q to which any reasonable person must subscribe. Now Popper would allow that it is quite possible for A's conjecture to be shown to be false (or highly probably to be false). Is it then not inevitably the case that B's hypothesis would automatically thereby be shown true (or highly probable to be true)?!
Once more the wise words of Dr. Johnson seem relevant:

The *irregular* combination of *fanciful* invention may delight awhile, by that *novelty* of which the *common satiety of life* send us all in quest; but the pleasures of sudden wonder are soon *exhausted*, and *the mind can only repose on the stability of the truth*.[4]

The sagacious Samuel Johnson would have sympathized with those who are thrilled with novelties like the thesis that scientific method is basically determined by the whimsies of paradigm-mongers, that induction is irrational, that in logic anything goes, etc. For a while, but for a while only, saith the good Doctor reassuringly, fanciful inventions of this kind may delight the mind questing for titillation. Ultimately, however, such sudden wonders are bound to lose their allurement. Would that he was not too optimistic about human nature!

References

1. Poincaré H. *The Value of Science.* New York: Dover, 1958:8.

2. Kermode F, ed. *The Selected Prose of T.S. Eliot.* New York: Harcourt, Brace & Jovanovich, 1975:97.

3. Lucas JR. *Space, Time and Causality.* Oxford: Oxford University Press, 1984:119.

4. The Rambler, No. 142.

Error and Uncertainty in Causal Inference

Stephan F. Lanes

Epidemiology Resources Inc.
Chestnut Hill, Massachusetts

I am uneasy to think I approve of one object, and disapprove of another; call one thing beautiful, and another deformed; decide concerning truth and falsehood, reason and folly, without knowing upon what principles I proceed.
David Hume[1]

The history of public health shows clearly the value of etiologic research in the prevention and treatment of disease. It was not long ago that we were virtually helpless in our fight against diseases such as smallpox, polio, cholera and syphilis. Today, thanks in large measure to our research efforts, we have learned a great deal about how to control these and many other diseases.

Although we take pride in our success, we know that history also will record our failures. Misadventures such as thalidomide and diethylstilbestrol (DES) serve as painful reminders that, despite our best efforts, we sometimes make mistakes. In expressing concern that several attempts to reduce the incidence of cholera actually had the opposite effect, John Snow[2] urged that "[t]he measures which are intended to prevent disease should be founded on a correct knowledge of its causes." In this spirit, we have made it our aim in epidemiology to establish an exposure as a cause of disease before we take preventive action. To this end, we have employed such methods as criteria of causality.

Everyone seems to agree that it is a good idea to interpret our results with caution. It is important, however, to temper our caution with the realizations that science is fallible and that we have to act, one way or another. Although we can learn to avoid certain kinds of mistakes, we should not forget that there is no way of avoiding mistakes entirely. My concern is that we do not become so cautious that we let our uncertainty interfere with our efforts to prevent disease. It is from this perspective of the tension between the need to act in public health and the unattainability of certainty in public health science that I have offered criticism of causal criteria.

My critics, for the most part, claim that I have somehow overlooked the application of epidemiologic research to public health problems.[3,4] If I understand this argument correctly, it reflects a misunderstanding of my views. If there were some way to establish that we had hit upon the truth, it would be foolish to suggest that we should not establish a causal relation before we decide to implement a policy aimed at preventing the disease in question. My point, however, is that we cannot know we are right. It is one thing to have looked for errors and to have found none; it is another thing to say that no errors exist to be found. My view is that time spent trying to confirm that which cannot be confirmed can only impede the application of useful ideas.

The response from some of my colleagues tells me that I did not succeed in expressing my views clearly. Nevertheless, I find considerable agreement in the notion that testing theories plays an essential role in eliminating mistakes in causal inference. The disagreement concerns the role that causal criteria play in this process, and whether or not interpretation requires methods above and beyond those necessary for the testing of theories. In an effort to clarify the arguments, I shall begin my rejoinder by restating my view of the problem of causal inference and the contribution empirical tests can make toward solving that problem. I shall try to make explicit the intellectual norms that have guided epidemiologists through critical contrasts of competing explanations, and I shall describe these standards as implicit rules of interpretation. I shall do so not with the intention of presenting anything new, but simply of establishing some common ground in the hope of separating areas of agreement more sharply from areas of disagreement.

The Problem of Causal Inference

The goal of an etiologic study is to find out whether a particular exposure causes a particular disease. In this sense, validity is qualitative: either a causal relation exists or it does not. We can say that causation (or prevention) is indicated by a valid observation that exposure increases (or decreases) the rate of disease occurrence. The problem of causal inference, therefore, lies in assessing the validity of observations that measure the effect of an exposure on the occurrence of a disease.

Falsification: The Search for Error

An association between exposure and disease may be distorted by several kinds of error. Errors can be made, for instance, by characterizing subjects incorrectly with respect to relevant exposures, by measuring inaccurately the occurrence of disease, or by not taking into account the effects of determinants of disease other than the exposure under study. If we could show that no errors were made, then causal inference would be certain. Since we cannot demonstrate that an association is valid, it is always possible that we have made an error. This possibility does not cause us undue concern, however. If the mere possibility of error were sufficient grounds to reject a study as invalid, then all studies would have to be rejected. As Cornfield[5] said, "If we ask for proof in medicine, or any other empirical science, we may be asking for something that does not exist." In recognition of our fallibility, epidemiologists have relied implicitly on the following "rule" of interpretation:

Rule 1:

We cannot infer that an association is noncausal merely because error is possible. For an error to be considered as a potential explanation of an association, there needs to be some way of evaluating whether or not an error did in fact occur.

It is not unusual for errors to occur, and when they do interpretation requires additional guidelines. Consider the observation that exposure to vaginal spermicides increased the prevalence of certain congenital anomalies from 1.0% to 2.2%.[6] In this study, fetuses were classified as exposed if the mother filled a prescription for spermicides at a large health maintenance organization within 600 days of delivery. It is clear that women who obtained spermicides may not have used them. Recently, it was shown that among eight infants with congenital anomalies who were classified as exposed, only four mothers actually used spermicides at or after the time of conception.[7] If spermicides could produce a teratogenic effect only if used at or after the time of conception, then the exposure characterization was, as one of the investigators put it, "grossly inaccurate."[7] Mounting doubts concerning the validity of the study prompted two of the investigators to acknowledge that they now feel the results do not indicate that a causal relation exists.[7,8]

Several co-investigators expressed a different interpretation.[9] They noted that exposure status had been reviewed for the cases of birth defects, but not for the non-cases. Since exposure status was originally determined from pharmacy records, the frequency of exposure misclassification should have been the same for the non-cases as it was for the cases. If so, and exposure misclassification was "nondifferential" or "random," the observed association was an *underestimate* of the effect of spermicides.[10] In fact, the more grossly inaccurate the exposure classification was, the greater was the underestimation of the teratogenic effect of spermicides. Demonstrating that an error exists, therefore, does not mean the association is qualitatively invalid. We need a second rule to prevent a study from being dismissed simply because an error was made:

Rule 2:

We cannot infer that an association is noncausal because a source of error is identified. We must determine the direction of bias, if any, that the error produced. A bias that diminishes an association cannot be considered an adequate explanation for an observed association.

As helpful as these two rules may be, they will not resolve the most difficult problems of interpretation. In the 1970s a controversy emerged regarding the relation between exogenous estrogens taken by post-menopausal women and the occurrence of endometrial cancer. Several studies reported that women who took these drugs experienced a rate of endometrial cancer that was many times higher than the rate among women who did not take estrogens.[11-14] Of the 67 cases of endometrial cancer that were observed in one study, for instance, 60 cases were seen among women taking estrogen when only five cases would have been expected if these women had experienced the same rate as the unexposed women (relative risk (RR) = 60/5 = 12).[14] It was suggested, however, that estrogens caused vaginal bleeding and that vaginal bleeding would make estrogen-users seek diagnostic tests.[15] A woman who developed asymptomatic endometrial cancer, therefore, would come to diagnosis more readily if she began taking estrogens. As a result of this hypothesized bias, we would observe an association between estrogens and endometrial cancer even if there were no causal relation. The bias was evaluated by examining autopsy records to identify women who had endometrial cancer at the time of death but whose disease had not been previously diagnosed.[15] The number of undiagnosed cases was compared with the number of women diagnosed with the disease during life, as estimated by the incidence rate from the Connecticut tumor registry, providing a ratio of undiagnosed cases to diagnosed cases of about 4:1.[15] These data showed that some cases of endometrial cancer are undiagnosed, and suggested to some researchers that the observed associations were invalid.

Subsequently, it was pointed out that an error had been made in evaluating the bias.[16,17] The *annual* risk from the tumor registry had been inappropriately compared with the *lifetime* risk as determined from autopsy data. To calculate the lifetime risk of being diagnosed with endometrial cancer, the proportion of cases occurring in one year would have to be multiplied by 35 years or more (assuming that endometrial cancer does not occur until age 35 and that the average lifespan is 70 years). Correcting for this error reveals that the ratio of undiagnosed to diagnosed cases should be approximately 1:4 instead of 4:1.[16,17] Thus, about 20% of the cases of endometrial cancer are undiagnosed during life. As a result of the detection bias, one should see about 20% more cases among estrogen-users than would otherwise be expected according to the rate at which endometrial cancer is diagnosed among women not taking estrogens. To quantify the effect of the bias in the aforementioned study,[14] let us assume that all of the women with undiagnosed disease took estrogens, and that all such cases became diagnosed for this reason. Five cases were expected among the estrogen users based on the rate among the unexposed women in the study. In consideration of the detection bias, we would see approximately two additional cases who became diagnosed because they took estrogens. To correct the estimated effect of estrogens for this bias, we would subtract the two cases observed because of the detection bias from the total number of cases observed among women taking estrogens: $RR_{corrected} = (60-2)/5 = 11.6$. Therefore, despite the fact that some cases of endometrial cancer are undiagnosed, there are not enough undiagnosed cases to explain the association observed in this study. This example illustrates the need for a third rule:

Rule 3:
We cannot infer that an association is noncausal because a source of error exists that would exert a bias in the direction of creating an association. To explain an association, the bias must be of sufficient magnitude to create the association that was observed.

I wish to emphasize that the three "rules" are intended simply to make explicit the thinking that epidemiologists have used to resolve some difficult problems of interpretation. Although each of us occasionally may not follow these principles, especially in the midst of a heated discussion, I think that all of us would agree to their merit.

The first rule draws a distinction between the possibility of error and the existence of error. In consideration of error introduced by the possibility of a confounding variable, Sir Austin Bradford Hill said:

> If we cannot detect [a confounding variable] or reasonably infer a specific one, then we are entitled to reject the vague contention of the armchair critic "you can't prove it, there *may* be such a feature."[18]

Indeed, if we did not accept the first rule demanding that an error be testable, we would have to surrender our results to the mere possibility of error and we would learn nothing from epidemiologic research.

The second and third rules extend the assessment of the effect of an error to include the direction and magnitude of its bias. Although the ultimate question of the existence of a causal relation is qualitative, the question of whether there is enough bias to explain a particular association is a quantitative problem. When this distinction is not recognized, studies may be dismissed before the effect of a bias has been assessed. In the spermicide study,[6] the second rule raises the question of the direction of the bias, which depends on whether or not exposure misclassification was nondifferential. The interpretive dilemma can be resolved by examining the exposure histories of the non-cases. In the endometrial cancer example, the direction of the detection bias was clear and the ratio of undiagnosed cases to diagnosed cases was estimated, but the magnitude of the bias was not calculated. For at least one study,[14] the magnitude of the bias was not large enough to explain the observed association. The third rule reminds us that studies containing enough bias to produce even a strong association nevertheless may be sufficiently accurate to show that an effect exists.

Verification: The Search for Validity

If we observe the three rules for interpreting empirical tests of competing explanations, we may sometimes find that we have eliminated as noncausal explanations all of the sources of error that we have been able to identify. Since we may not have identified all of the sources of error, however, the three rules can never establish that an association is causal. We employ causal criteria in an attempt to bridge this gap, as Cole explains:

Occasionally, the causal inference is made as "a diagnosis of exclusion." That is, if the result is not perceived as biased and not due to chance or confounding, then it must be causal. But causality has positive criteria and these should be reviewed, *in addition to excluding alternative explanations*.[19] (emphasis added)

Similarly, it is only Doll's[20] *first* requirement for establishing causality that an association "is not explicable by bias in recording or detection, confounding or chance." If, after careful scrutiny, we cannot find a bias capable of explaining an association, Doll offers additional criteria that, if met, would provide "positive" evidence that the association is causal.

Criteria of "positive" evidence can be viewed in terms of error-elimination, as several contributors to this monograph have pointed out.[4,21,22] Semantics aside, however, there is a real distinction to be made. The three rules of "negative" evidence help us evaluate the sources of error that have been specifically identified. Once we have controlled for all the sources of error we have been able to identify, the only obstacle standing in the way of our being certain that a result is valid is the possibility that there still exists a source of error that we have not identified. The notion of positive evidence, therefore, refers to unspecified sources of error.

Causal inference is uncertain, of course, so causal criteria cannot *eliminate* the possibility of bias due to an unspecified source of error. Rather, causal criteria are intended to help us evaluate the *likelihood* of bias due to an unspecified error. This probabilistic view of validity is apparent in the question posed by Hill[18] in presenting his criteria: "What aspects of [an] association should we consider before deciding that the *most likely* interpretation of it is causation?" (emphasis added)

Consider, for example, the strength of an association as a probabilistic indicator of causality. We have this criterion despite the general appreciation that a strong association (RR $\gg$ 1) may be noncausal and that a weak association may be causal. We know, however, that in order for a confounding variable to explain an association, it would have to be associated with the disease at least as strongly as the exposure under study. Reasoning further, Susser states:

Very strong relationships are much less common than weak ones in epidemiological analysis. Thus the stronger the relationship, the less a confounding variable capable of explaining the association is likely to exist.[21]

In other words, a stronger association is *less likely* than a weaker association to result solely from the effect of an unspecified confounding variable.[18,21,22]

Let us examine more closely the statement, "Strong associations are more likely to be causal than weak associations." To make probabilistic inferences of this kind, we would need to know something about the universe, or sample space, to which the inference applies.[23] Everyone who has taken a statistics course has heard about an urn containing so many red balls and so many blue balls. The probability of drawing from the urn a ball of a particular color depends on the distribution of different colored balls in the urn. In the case of causal criteria, the "urn" is the universe of all possible associations between exposures and diseases, causal and noncausal.

If we are to view an observed association as a sample from the universe of all associations, our first task would be to try to identify the sample space. Although it is not clear how this undertaking could be accomplished, let us assume that we have not only identified all possible associations, but that we have also established that within this universe strong associations are less common than weak associations. It still does not follow that a strong association is more likely to be causal. Whatever the proportions of strong and weak associations may be, we would need to know that the proportion of causal relations is greater among strong associations than among weak associations. Suppose that we could enumerate each sample space comprising every strong association and every weak association; how would we determine which associations in each group were causal? We cannot point to a list of "established" causal associations to evaluate causal criteria because associations appear on these lists by virtue of having met causal criteria. Yet, if we had a better method than causal criteria to serve as the standard for determining which associations were causal, we would have no need for the criteria in the first place.

Since there is no method of identifying causal associations, we cannot know the proportions of strong and weak associations that are causal. The statement, "Strong associations are more likely to be causal than weak associations" can be supported by the facts no better and no worse than contradictory statements, such as, "Weak associations are more likely to be causal than strong associations," or "Weak associations and strong associations are equally likely to be causal." The strength-of-association criterion, like other causal criteria, is an untestable tautology.

It is often argued that Hill did not intend for these criteria to be hard and fast rules, and that we should view causal criteria as viewpoints,[18] or as criteria of judgment.[24] This subtle shift to subjectivism, while creating many problems of its own, does not touch upon my criticism. By adopting a subjective interpretation of probability, we shift the object of interpretation from our theories about the causation of disease to our personal beliefs. Under the subjective view, causal criteria do not tell us whether an exposure causes disease. Instead, they tell us which characteristics of epidemiologic associations "help us make up our minds" about causality.[18] The problem, however, is not that I fail to grasp the distinction between theory and belief, as Greenland[4] claims; the problem is that our subjective beliefs do not constitute anything in the way of evidentiary support for a causal theory. The difficulty with causal criteria remains: there is no reason to think they are true and, more importantly, there is no way to discover if they are false.

   To summarize this argument, everyone seems to agree that causal criteria cannot tell us with certainty that an association is causal. We also find, perhaps more surprisingly, that they cannot even tell us that an association is probably causal. Since there is no way to calculate the probability that a scientific theory is true or false, there is no way to calculate the probability that an exposure causes a disease.[1] It follows that there can be no empirical support for the conclusion that causation is the "most likely" explanation for any association. In short, there can be no "positive" evidence to support the claim that an association is valid.[1,25] If this conclusion disturbs us, we need only recall that causal criteria are intended to overcome uncertainty due to the possibility of unspecified sources of error. Without specifying the source of an error, however, there is no way to determine whether the error occurred. To discredit an association on the basis of an error that cannot be demonstrated would be to violate our first rule of interpretation.

   The quest for validity, combined with the demand that an error be testable (rule 1), creates a conflict that spells trouble not only for causal criteria, but for the "chance explanation" as well. "Chance" refers to a distribution of observations under a probability model. Probability models answer problems that require probabilistic solutions, such as the likelihood of tossing a "one" with a particular die. The answer to a probability problem is a probability, such as 1/6. Probability models cannot tell us *why* we might see statistical regularity; they simply assert that certain experimental conditions will, if repeated, produce a particular distribution of results. The important thing about a probability model, as with any hypothesis, is whether it is right or wrong. Probability models should be testable empirically by seeing whether a group of observations conforms to the probability model. If the observations do not conform to the probability model from which we are supposed to be sampling, we will question the validity of the model. Thus, if we want to know whether a die is loaded, we must toss the die many times in a certain way. If, upon repeated tosses of the die, the number "one" does not appear with a frequency of about 1/6, we may suspect that the die is loaded and, therefore, that the probability model we have chosen is incorrect. The question of whether an occurrence of disease was caused by a particular exposure is not a probabilistic question.[26] Nevertheless, the view that an association can be attributed to chance appears to require that probability models be appended to causal hypotheses. The thoughtful scientist may wonder, "What is chance?"[4] Attempts to answer this question point to a fundamental problem. In their typical application, probability models assert that if exposure does not cause disease (i.e., if the "null" hypothesis is true), and we have eliminated the effects of the sources of error we have identified (i.e., if there is no apparent bias), we still may observe an association. If exposure does not cause disease, however, and we observe an association, then our observation is in error. If the association is not created by an error that we have identified, it would have to be due to an error that has not been identified. Indeed, the popular view is that chance represents the effects of factors about which we are ignorant.[1,4,24,27] Rothman[28] expresses succinctly this notion that chance "is that part of our experience that we cannot predict."

I recognize, of course, that few things can be predicted with certainty, and I will not quibble if we want to refer to our ignorance as chance. What I find troublesome is the assertion that the effects of errors that cannot be demonstrated and, therefore, may not exist, somehow can be predicted to obey the laws of probability. I do not claim that this assertion is false. I merely wish to point out that any statement about the existence of an unspecified source of error is untestable[29] and, therefore, inadmissible in causal inference if we are to abide by the first rule of interpretation.

The lack of testability of probability models in epidemiology has important implications for their interpretation. It is always possible to append a probability model to an observed association and calculate statistical p-values. These p-values, however, have an objective interpretation only insofar as the observation can be viewed as a sample from a group of observations. Whether we are drawing balls from an urn or repeatedly tossing a die, the sampling variability is the variation in the sample space.

What has become the conventional practice of calculating p-values for an epidemiologic measure of effect follows from the premise that in the absence of randomization study subjects are drawn at random from some sort of imaginary superpopulation. The key point here is that there is no empirical sample space. As Robins and Morgenstern[30] put it, "the superpopulation model is a fiction." I do not see how an empirical interpretation of sampling variability can be deduced from a sample space that does not exist. Although it is often said that study subjects "are always a sample,"[28] I concur with Miettinen[31] that, in causal inference, "there is no point in trying to make the study experience a probability sample." In claiming that there can be no objective interpretation of sampling variability when there is no sampling, I side completely with the subjectivists in their criticism of conventional practice. I do not share their interest in subjective interpretations of probability, however, because as an epidemiologist I am interested in the causes of disease, as opposed to the causes of belief, and, insofar as subjective probability statements pertain to the causes of disease, these statements, like causal criteria, are untestable.[29]

Conclusion

Very few philosophers or scientists still think that scientific knowledge is, or can be proven knowledge. But few realize that with this the classical structure of intellectual values falls in ruins and has to be replaced: one cannot simply water down the ideal of proven truth to the ideal of "probable truth" or to "truth by (changing) consensus."
Imre Lakatos[32]

The uncertainty in causal inference is attributable to the fact that we cannot establish that an association is valid. It is always possible that we have made an error. Moreover, an unidentifiable error cannot be assessed by causal criteria, statistical probability, or any other methodology. We can never know if an unidentifiable error exists or, if it does, whether it produced our observation.

The upshot is that solutions to the problem of causal inference get off to a bad start with the aim of establishing causality. The goal of justifying causal relations leads to a subjective framework in which error cannot be distinguished from uncertainty. This distinction is crucial because, although it is possible to get rid of error, proof is unattainable and uncertainty inevitable. Any attempt to overcome uncertainty will be influenced by features of the data that affect subjective beliefs but that have nothing to do with validity, such as the strength of an association, the shape of a dose-response curve, or the level of statistical significance. Consequently, the view that causal inference is a matter of opinion disuades us from explaining our observations. For example, even if studies showing no association between spermicides and birth defects are valid and plentiful, they do not support the popular opinion that the "overwhelming body of medical evidence indicates that spermicides are not teratogenic."[33-35] What is called for are (noncausal) explanations of the effects that have been reported.[6,36,37] This kind of mistake can be avoided by following the three rules of interpretation.

Causal inference should be motivated by a search for error. The first principle of interpretation requires that an error be testable for it to qualify as a possible explanation of an association. To the extent that we concern ourselves with uncertainty instead of error, observation yields inevitably to presupposition as the arbiter of our theories. The objective view rejects the traditional aim of causal inference, since even if we have eliminated as noncausal explanations all of the sources of error that we can identify, we will not have established that an association is causal. Perhaps the greatest lesson from the history of public health, however, is that we do not have to establish causality to prevent disease.

References

1. Hume D. *A Treatise of Human Nature.* London: John Noon, 1739; revised and reprinted, Selby-Bigge LA, ed. Oxford: Clarendon Press, 1985:Book 1, part iii, sections vi,xi,xii.

2. Snow J. *Snow On Cholera.* New York: Hafner Publishing Company, 1965:136.

3. Labarthe DR, Stallones RA. Epidemiologic inference. In this volume.

4. Greenland S. Probability versus Popper: An elaboration of the insufficiency of current Popperian approaches for epidemiologic analysis. In this volume.

5. Cornfield J. Statistical relationships and proof in medicine [Editorial]. Am Statistician 1954;8:19–21.

6. Jick H, Walker AM, Rothman KJ, et al. Vaginal spermicides and congenital disorders. JAMA 1981;245:1329–1332.

7. Watkins RN. The validity of a study [Letter]. JAMA 1986;256:3094–3095.

8. Holmes LB. The validity of a study [Letter]. JAMA 1986;256:3096.

9. Jick H, Walker AM, Rothman KJ, et al. The validity of a study [Letter]. JAMA 1986;256:3095–3096.

10. Copeland KT, Checkoway H, McMichael AJ, et al. Bias due to misclassification in the estimation of relative risk. Am J Epidemiol 1977;105:488–495.

11. Smith DC, Prentice R, Thompson DJ, et al. Association of exogenous estrogen and endometrial carcinoma. N Engl J Med 1975;293:1164–1167.

12. Gordon J, Reagan JW, Finkle WD, et al. Estrogen and endometrial carcinoma. N Engl J Med 1977;297:570–571.

13. Antunes CMF, Stolley PD, Rosenshein NB, et al. Endometrial cancer and estrogen use. N Engl J Med 1979;300:9–13.

14. Jick H, Watkins RN, Hunter JR, et al. Replacement estrogens and endometrial cancer. N Engl J Med 1979;300:218–222.

15. Horwitz RA, Feinstein AR, Horwitz SM, et al. Necropsy diagnosis of endometrial cancer and detection bias in case-control studies. Lancet 1981;2:66–68.

16. Crombie IK, Tomenson J. Detection bias in endometrial cancer [Letter]. Lancet 1981;2:308–309.

17. Merletti F, Cole P. Detection bias and endometrial cancer [Letter]. Lancet 1981;2:310–312.

18. Hill AB. The environment and disease: Association or causation? Proc Roy Soc Med 1965;58:295–300.

19. Cole P. Introduction. In: Breslow NE, Day NE, eds. *Statistical methods in cancer research. I. The analysis of case-control studies.* Lyon: IARC Scientific Publications, 1980:36.

20. Doll R. Occupational cancer: A hazard for epidemiologists? Int J Epidemiol 1985;14:22–31.

21. Susser M. Falsification, verification and causal inference in epidemiology: Reconsiderations in the light of Sir Karl Popper's Philosophy. In this volume.

22. Maclure M. Refutation in epidemiology: Why else not? In this volume.

23. Freedman D, Pisani R, Purves R. *Statistics.* New York: W.W. Norton & Company, 1978:407,497.

24. Susser M. *Causal Thinking in the Health Sciences.* New York: Oxford University Press, 1973:140,136.

25. Popper K, Miller D. A proof of the impossibility of inductive probability [Letter]. Nature 1983;21:687–688.

26. Popper KR. *The Logic of Scientific Discovery.* Revised ed. New York: Harper & Row, 1968:254–270. Originally published as *Logik der Forschung.* Vienna: Springer, 1934.

27. Kleinbaum DG, Kupper LL, Morgenstern H. *Epidemiologic Research.* Belmont, California: Lifetime Learning Publications, 1982:37.

28. Rothman KJ. *Modern Epidemiology.* Boston: Little, Brown and Company, 1986:78.

29. Popper KR. Probability magic or knowledge out of ignorance. Dialectica 1957;11:354–374.

30. Robins JM, Morgenstern H. The statistical foundations of confounding in epidemiology. Computers and Mathematics with Application (in press), 1987.

31. Miettinen OS. *Theoretical Epidemiology.* New York: John Wiley & Sons, 1985:47.

32. Lakatos I. Falsification and the methodology of scientific research programs. In: Lakatos I, Musgrave A, eds. *Criticism and the Growth of Knowledge.* London: Cambridge University Press, 1984:92.

33. Mills JL, Alexander D. Teratogens and "Litogens" [Editorial]. N Engl J Med 1986;315:1234–1236.

34. FDA Drug Bulletin 1986;16(2):21.

35. Shapiro S. Oral-contraceptive use and the risk of breast cancer [Letter]. N Engl J Med 1987;316:164.

36. Strobino B, Kline J, Lai A, et al. Vaginal spermicides and spontaneous abortion of known karyotype. Am J Epidemiol 1986;123:431–433.

37. Rothman KJ. Spermicides and Down's syndrome. Am J Public Health 1982;72:399–401.

Rational Science Versus a System of Logic

Mervyn Susser

Gertrude H. *Sergievsky Center*
Columbia University

Plato is the apotheosis of high seriousness. One of his dialogues having been named a *symposium*, this word for a convivial gathering for conversation, or a report of such exchanges, then acquired its present graver sense. This response to the critics of my paper "Falsification and Verification . . ." harks back to the origins of the word, and may appear to some light, to others sharp. Nonetheless, I respond to protect rationality in the manner of science, and pragmatism in the manner of a goal-oriented discipline like epidemiology. Arguments such as these may have material consequences both for the quality of our work and for the public weal.

Here I respond only to those symposiasts who seem to me in danger of propagating a Popperian ideology rather than a philosophy of science, and mostly to McIntyre and Poole, who are my direct critics. I am a practitioner of science who has learned from Popper but does not follow him. Thus I have preferred a "hypothetico-deductive" style, and frequently my results have clashed with received wisdom. Yet I do not recognize, in the propositions of these writers, the lineaments of my long-time scientific activity.

Karl Popper himself must be accorded the standing of a major figure in the contemporary philosophy of science. To reduce his arduous thought to a few key elements is presumptuous, but necessary to my purpose of contrasting and comparing Popper's philosophy with the ideology of Popperians. In doing so, I draw mainly on Popper's *Logic of Scientific Discovery* and on some commentators on Popper. Popper's avowed concern, aptly expressed in the title of what was his first major work published in English, is with the *logic* of scientific discovery.[1] His actual concerns go well beyond that. The logic is ensconced within and constrained by a philosophical *system*. We need to distinguish between the logical procedures advocated by Popper and the philosophical system in which he embeds those procedures, a system that has broad implications.

Popper introduced a new and appealing criterion for separating science from non-science. In Popper's terms, the demarcation lies in the capacity of science to pose potentially testable hypotheses. Science, as Peter Medawar put it more narrowly, is the art of the soluble. Of course Popper did not, as some commentators in this book may allow readers to think, invent the procedure of "strong inference," that is, testing tightly drawn hypotheses. Popper is not unique either in preferring deduction to induction. He *is* original, as far as I know, in putting verification out of court on logical grounds, in relying solely on the refutation of hypotheses in the pursuit of truth, and in developing a consistent philosophy around these issues.

Popper came to dismiss induction by way of the arguments of David Hume. Like Plato and George Berkeley who epitomize idealist philosophy, Hume constructed a view of the world that gives primacy to the sentience and thought of the individual: truth can be said to exist only in the subjective perceptions of an observer. For Hume the "apparent sequence of events in the external world is in fact the sequence of perceptions in the mind." He could find no basis in *reason* for the expectation that the future will be like the past: that a stone will fall, or fire burn, was for him a matter of belief. Samuel Johnson's refutation of Hume was that he knew a rock because he could kick it. Another critic expressed himself in a limerick:

There was a young man who said God
Must find it exceedingly odd
That this tree
Continues to be
When there's no one about in the quad.

In fact Hume, unlike some of Popper's followers, conceded that theoretical skepticism is irrelevant to the practical concerns of daily life. He recognized that "nature is always too strong for principle," and that no durable good could arise from excessive skepticism.

Popper himself I think also differs in this matter from his followers in this book. Popper says that ". . . in spite of the 'rationality' of choosing the best-tested theory as a basis of action, the choice is *not* 'rational' in the sense that it is based upon *good reasons* for expecting that it will in practice be a successful choice...."[2] While he is saying that in logic the choice is rational, he admits at the same time that in practice such a choice eschews rationality. Like Hume, Popper concedes to the real world when he says further that a pragmatic belief in the results of science is not irrational. (The belief is justified, he holds, because there is nothing more rational than the method of critical discussion. The weighing of results and knowledge, I may add, seems to me to entail induction.)

Popper's search for a consistent logic in science, coupled with his rejection of induction, thus divorces the logic of science from the practice of science. Popper's implicit dichotomy between philosophy and practical reality must surely be crucial for an epidemiologist. Indeed, it has obliged some contributors, as Labarthe and Stallones observe, to separate the domains of science and action, or to ignore action, in order to escape epidemiological paralysis. In this lies the fundamental issue on which Popper challenges vulgar, commonsensical, and pragmatic materialists like myself. Materialists, and Popper too, accord primacy to the material world—which includes Popper's World III of culture and society—and consider their perceptions to be shaped by that world. At this point I depart from Popper. However dependent all may be on sentience, and uncertain about what is true, the material world is there to be acted upon and understood. It is to be understood from the cumulation, in history and in our individual life-cycles, of multifarious cross-referenced interactions with the world. As Dr. Johnson implied, it is *verified* by the demonstrable consequences of our activity.

McIntyre seems to have an intuition that he has been led into a cul-de-sac. As a physician, he must make diagnoses and act upon them to pursue his clinical functions. Presumably for that reason he wishes to allow the possibility, antithetical to Popper's logical system, that a diagnosis can be *confirmed*. He achieves this license, I fear, by verbal sleight of hand: in confirming a diagnosis, he argues, he is confirming only a definition or a classification. Thus, he disconnects his definition from reality, since the disorder being named does not "exist in its own right." Doubtless a cure for a serious disease requires no more than reassigning it to a classification for minor illness.

It is not clear to me that all the epidemiological disciples of Popper, unlike Popper himself, fully appreciate the conflict about reality that underlies the ancient controversy between idealism and materialism. Certainly one does not need philosophical systems like those of Berkeley, Hume or Popper to arrive at a skeptical and critical stance. For verification—or should I say for refutation—we need look no further than to the archmaterialists Karl Marx and Friedrich Engels. Popper himself is a radical skeptic. A pervasive problem among Popperian ideologues is that they themselves too readily abandon his skepticism. Where is their vaunted rational criticism when they examine Popper's philosophy? Nowhere do I find a hint that Popper could speak anything but the hallowed truth.

Arguments against opposing views are mostly dealt with by such devices as counterassertions, appeals to authority, semantic fencing, or neglect. For instance, a scientist may claim to be making a general statement about probabilies by induction from a sample. Our commentators indicate that they would be bold enough to say they know better: the truth is that the scientist is making a deduction from an implicit general model, one which he has in mind whether he knows it or not. And if the reader should remain skeptical, they cite this or that authority (as Poole cites Cox and Hinkley on this very point). In this matter of probability, Poole invents a statistical parable to illustrate Popper's deductive approach. He concludes the parable with a *non sequitur*, the assertion that "no probability statement, inside or outside of epidemiology, is an inductive generalization from a sample to a population." An innocent would never guess that, from the moment Thomas Bayes invented the theory of probability to the present day, the inductive approach has been explicated in major works in philosophy and statistics.

With meager equipment in the field, I am in no position to contest Popper or any other authority in a matter of probability theory. Yet it seems to me that Popper's central concern is to achieve the conformity of his probability theory with his system of logic. In the course of the arguments in which he reveals this concern, he also concedes that the scientific *use* of probability may not conform with his conception of the *logic* of probability. Thus he does not rule out induction in arriving at probability statements when he says that "I do not see any reason why such conjectures should be inspired *only* (my italics) by the accumulation of a large mass of inductive observations" (*The Logic of Scientific Discovery*, page 169). And although he holds that probability hypotheses are not falsifiable and do not rule out anything observable, he allows that in practice if not in logic we would abandon an estimate that was many times contradicted (*Logic of Scientific Discovery*, page 190ff). Indeed, in a footnote (page 191) he goes so far as to admit "the fact that probability statements are . . . in some sense verifiable. . . ." Ultimately, he finds that a "methodological rule" is essential to reconcile his theory of probability with the practical efficiency of probability statements. Thus to reach a decision, some minimum standard of *agreement* between hypothesis and observed facts is needed.

The truth seems to be, then, that here induction has after all been admitted into Troy. For epidemiologists, in any case, abstruse theory is beside the point. I venture that no casino owners anywhere have used a deductive approach. They have had no need of a prior statistical model to estimate probabilities and ensure their profits at the gaming tables. Without so much as a nod toward deduction, they work all the time from a sample to a population (which is to say by induction from the particular to the general) and virtually never fail.

Again, if a scientist denies he has a theory—indeed, if he is totally ignorant of the field he enters—Popperian ideologues will trick him out with a theory improvised from his prejudices, biases, premonitions, and "vague expectations." This is accomplished by having the idea that concepts and preconceptions guide our choice of problems and our understanding of cause— an idea that I too have expounded for at least 25 years[3,4]—stand in for real theory. No matter that Popper demands logic and rationality above all. The scientist may follow the practice of centuries in requiring that a theory should reflect a coherent structure of thought and ideas, or he may follow Popper in believing that a scientific theory must have sufficient content to be testable, but if he denies he has such a theory, they insist on fitting him out with one from such rags and patches as they can find.

While this psychological technique might serve on the psychoanalyst's couch, it will not do in the rational world of logic, science and the actual. Least of all should it do in Popper's own view. Sigmund Freud's fertile construct of the unconscious, a psychodynamics by definition hidden from the individual, was strongly criticized by Popper. As he saw it, the theory defied testing because circularity of thought ensued from it. The psychoanalyst could always transform the literal facts of his subject's talk and behavior by resort to their metamorphosis, in the subject's unconscious, into their opposites.

Popper is puritanical about "the avoidance of verbal issues" in his pursuit of logic, but not his disciples. McIntyre finesses the issue of induction and verification, in support of Popper's position, with a quibble about my shorthand use of "deduction" instead of the "hypothetico-deductive" system explained in my next sentence. (McIntyre also alleges that "Susser considers . . . a statistically significant result affirms the hypothesis," an allegation which surprised me. I do describe such a result as "affirmative," that is, having a tendency to affirm. We do indeed use the same words to mean different things, as he suggests.) He goes on to ask,

While Susser may remember results that have been incompatible with the truth of a given hypothesis, can he quote any which could be said to have verified or to have *proved* the hypothesis? . . . I suspect not; instead the results would have been considered to have strengthened the hypothesis. . . .

   McIntyre's second sentence seems to me to contradict the intent of the first. Popper would probably not admit the second as legitimate, since it conveys an affirmatory stance compatible with mine. Still, the first sentence—a challenge to my logic, if also to my memory and my knowledge—deserves an answer.

   The challenge can be framed in a simple example. Besides refuting the hypothesis that the earth is flat, can we not affirm that it is spherical? To naysayers we may retort, did Magellan circumnavigate the world, or did he and his shipmates cook the results of the voyage of 1519-22? And what of the thousands who have followed under sail or steam or on the wing? In *de Motu Cordis* (1628), William Harvey established the circulation of the blood to the continuing satisfaction of anatomists of the past three centuries and more. In *Haemostaticks* (1733), Stephen Hale demonstrated the phenomenon of blood pressure to the equal satisfaction of physiologists of the past two centuries and more. Do Popperians, whether philosophers or ideologues, doubt Theodore Schwann (*Structure of Plants and Animals*, 1846) and Virchow (*Cellular Pathology as Based on Histology*, 1856) on the cellularity of the body? Or James Watson and Francis Crick on the helical structure of DNA?

   I suppose that Popper would assign such well-established knowledge to the category of basic statements. These examples of background knowledge in no need of testing are nonetheless examples of verification. They have served practicing scientists as well as any falsification. By contrast, the research program recommended by McIntyre, based on "a constant search for errors," can only be sterile. Petitti, who reports a conversion experience to Popperism, should take care that she is not led out of one desert and into another. The true spirit of science is positive. The building of theory is art; it depends on imaginative synthesis, most often by inductive sifting, sometimes by a leap of the mind. The execution of tests (either falsification or verification) is craft; it depends on ingenuity and technique. The refutation of the theory of spontaneous generation was sealed by Louis Pasteur's verification of the positive role of bacteria in fermentation (1862). Much earlier Spallanzini, and then Schulze, Schwann and others, had refuted the theory when they showed that under controlled conditions fermentation did not occur.[5] Falsification was less successful here than verification because supporters of the theory could advance an endless series of alternative explanations. It is Pasteur's work that is remembered, whether justly or not.

Poole begins with semantic pyrotechnics and what I suspect is hyperbole; one supposes that he intends to pull beards. He disputes "that any characteristic of an exposure-disease association can make it objectively more or less likely to be causal." Schlesinger has reminded us of Cicero's despair that "there is nothing so absurd but that some philosopher has said it." With his single cavalier assertion, Poole proscribes most of modern epidemiological research. What possible point might there then be in unconfounding, refining, specifying, strengthening, elaborating, and clarifying any association once it has been observed for the first time. All these activities yield characteristics of associations that change our initial perceptions of them and their causal potential. Since I have dealt with these matters at length in one of my books,[4] there is no need to expand on them here. Poole espouses Popper's "rational critical discussion of causal theories" as "the best way of interpreting epidemiological research. . . ." Such discussion will carry us no distance at all without our better understanding of the characteristics of an observed association. Perhaps Poole is a thoroughgoing Berkeleyite, and has abandoned the notion of material causality.

A semantic maneuver settles the issue of induction for Poole. If you find you cannot do without induction to describe some of the scientific activity involved in generating an hypothesis, like Humpty Dumpty you may make a word mean just what you choose it to mean: if induction is not quite deduction but you wish it were, eliminate the problem by making it mean something in between. Elevate "vaguely formulated expectations" into theory, rename the inductive reasoning process "retroduction," and the transformation is accomplished. Is there an experienced epidemiologist who has not been humbled by ignorance of what causes or factors to consider in facing a totally obscure condition, and who has not been obliged to proceed from there by induction? Evidently, this has never happened to Poole. One has no doubt that it will.

Here I should perhaps confront Popper's system of logic with my understanding of the real world of science. Since for Popper induction is a mere myth and verification of a theory is never possible, he bases his system on the hypothetico-deductive method of falsification. This method is indeed powerful in rooting out error, but for Popper neither this method nor any other adds to the likely truth of a theory under test. In his system, since there are an infinity of alternatives, any future event is perfectly compatible with such evidence as we now have. (Hence, some followers of Popper, it seems, feel free to propose *any* theory.) I have never met and cannot imagine a productive scientist who *acts* on this assumption: any who did will have been dismissed as cranks.

What then is Popper's guide for action in science? In preferring one hypothesis or theory over others, he would go first by its simplicity (in his sense equivalent to falsifiability), and by its universality and precision (both of which add to falsifiability). He would choose it also for its verisimilitude, which is to say that among theories that survive testing it accounts for more instances of fact. The aim of science is to discover universal laws, the probability of a universal theory is zero, and it follows from this logical system that the best surviving theory for testing is the *most improbable*. Can there be an epidemiologist—indeed has there ever been one—who in his research program would choose a theory for testing on this ground? Can there be an epidemiologist, moreover, who would not choose a theory that has the highest probability of predicting "the next instance" (in accord with the proposition derived by Rudolf Carnap from inductive logic) rather than a universe of instances? If there is one, he has surely never been funded. Popper's immense intellectual effort to create a coherent logical system has led him to encourage choices among hypotheses that are more likely to retard than to advance science.

I repeat the position I stated in my initial symposium contribution. O'Hear[6] poses the issues well. Can it be denied that one is engaged in induction if one follows Popper's criteria and chooses, as a guide to further investigation or to policy, one theory among many—whether or not it is the best-tested or the most improbable? Moreover, if for the sake of argument one accepts Popper's position that one cannot choose among theories on the basis of their inductive probability—because there is no such thing and hence no way of recognizing their relative truth—what advantage for a scientist can one theory have over another? In the event, when Popper allows the scientist to choose among theories, he also allows induction to enter his system.

Some points of detail may bear mention. Austin Bradford Hill's classic paper of 1965[7] is not the first systematic naming, listing and discussion of criteria of judgment in causal inference currently in use. The first, if somewhat rudimentary, attempt I know of is to be found in the 1964 Report of the Advisory Committee to the Surgeon General on Smoking and Health.[8] Some asides from Poole also need to be put straight. He asserts three times that my arguments for induction "reiterate the claims of others" (namely those of Jacobsen and Davies in 1976). To this charge of unoriginality he adds one of shallowness. Thus, "great breadth and precious little depth . . ." typify papers on causal inference; and "Susser devotes no more than a paragraph to reiterating Jacobsen's and Davies' claims." Perhaps both charges can be attributed to the fact that my own fuller endeavors in this area echo from a receding past. No doubt I relied too heavily on my subtitle, namely, "Reconsiderations in the Light of Sir Karl Popper's Philosophy," by which I meant to indicate to readers that it led off from my own first consideration of these topics in my book of 1973.[4] While this was the first such book in epidemiology, it is so far also the last.

References

1. Popper KR. *The Logic of Scientific Discovery.* 2nd ed. New York: Harper & Row, 1968. Originally published as *Logik der Forschung.* Vienna: Springer, 1934.

2. Popper KR. *Objective Knowledge: Evolutionary Approach.* 1st ed. Oxford: Clarendon Press, 1972.

3. Susser M, Watson W. *Sociology in Medicine.* 1st ed. New York: Oxford University Press, 1962.

4. Susser M. *Causal Thinking in the Health Sciences: Concepts and Strategies in Epidemiology.* New York: Oxford University Press, 1973.

5. Winslow CEA. *The Conquest of Epidemic Disease: A Chapter in the History of Ideas.* Princeton, NJ: Princeton University Press, 1943; reprinted, Madison, Wisconsin: University of Wisconsin Press, 1980.

6. O'Hear A. *Karl Popper.* London: Routledge and Kegan Paul, 1980.

7. Hill AB. The environment and disease: association or causation. Proc Roy Soc Med 1965;58:1217–1219.

8. United States Department of Health, Education, and Welfare. Smoking and health: Report of the Advisory Committee to the Surgeon General. Washington, D.C.: Public Health Service, 1964.

Criticism and Its Constraints: A Self-Appraisal and Rejoinder

Douglas L. Weed

Biometry Branch
Division of Cancer Prevention and Control
National Cancer Institute
Bethesda, Maryland

It is not a sign of weakness...to rise to the level of self-criticism.
Martin Luther King, Jr.[1]

After reading the papers in this volume, I realize that those of us who delve into the philosophic basis of epidemiologic inference have only just scratched the surface of what could easily become a deep exploratory excavation. I also realize that any headway we make will depend upon the strength of the ideas we choose to illuminate our way. Judging again from these papers, the "Popperian" philosophy of critical rationalism provides us with a reasonably bright light. It has helped me to clarify my own thinking to such an extent that I consider it more a torch: the torch of criticism fueled by the pursuit of truth.

Criticism comes in many forms. It can be directed at one's own work or at the work of others. It can be constructive when it points out the errors in our solutions to problems and motivates us to suggest better ones. Criticism can also be destructive when it is used only to find our errors.[2] However it is used, criticism finds our mistakes. This should come easily to those who espouse some form of critical rationalism for epidemiology.

It is fundamental to this way of thinking that our mistakes teach us more than our successes.

We are in need of criticism's ability to uncover our mistakes for the simple reason that we have so much to learn; what we don't know far outweighs what we do know. In our ignorance, the pursuit of truth meets its nemesis.

Perhaps we should take our ignorance a little more seriously. In my contribution,[3] I acknowledge that I have introduced more problems than solutions. Furthermore, the solutions I have managed to eke out are incomplete, and to some extent, incorrect. I would be very surprised—even disappointed—if the other contributors to this volume, especially those who espouse some form of critical rationalism, would not admit to the same. After all, another key Popperian idea is that all knowledge, including any found in this volume, is conjectural, uncertain, tentative, and error-prone.

Fortunately, knowledge can also be improved. Improvements in methodologic knowledge occur, for example, when our solutions to new problems both explain and correct the errors in the solutions to our old problems.

In the spirit of this introduction, I take up where I left off and criticize my general solution to the problem of criteria for epidemiologic inference. In the course of this self-appraisal, I will also entertain some of the criticisms offered by other contributors to this volume.

Self-Criticism #1: Has Any Progress Been Made?

I begin by questioning whether the criteria of predictability and testability—suggested in my contribution to this volume[3]—represent progress in methodologic knowledge. How can they be better than the more familiar criteria? Specifically, how do they both explain earlier criteria and correct errors in them?

Before answering these questions, it is important to point out at least one of the errors that requires correction. Consider, for example, the following error of omission: lacking in many epidemiologic discussions of inferential criteria—including one[4] or two[5] in this volume—is a way to exploit the problem of theoretic diversity.

Causality is not a single simple notion. It enjoys a great variety of guises: a cause can be a sufficient condition, a necessary condition, a necessary and sufficient condition, a contributory or component condition, or an initial condition in a more general, biologic explanation, to name just a few. As if this weren't enough, we can easily add to this causal diversity the full range of noncausal hypotheses appropriate for epidemiologic inquiry, hypotheses such as those involving preventive agents, or those that explain selection processes.

One answer, then, to the questions posed above is that progress in methodologic knowledge can occur if a new approach is able to handle the theoretic diversity demonstrated by the full range of both causal and noncausal hypotheses.

The criterion of predictability does just that. It explicitly solves the problem of theoretic diversity because it is applicable to any sort of hypothesis we can come up with. To its credit, it also explains the dependency of many of Hill's original criteria upon specific hypotheses. Examples of such hypothesis-dependent criteria are consistency, the magnitude of an association, temporality, and biologic gradient.

But predictability is not a complete answer to my original question regarding progress; it alone is not sufficient. Somehow, predictions must also be linked to observation. The companion criterion of testability does just that. It cements the link between prediction and observation, by assuring that our predictions can either clash with observations, and be refuted, or match the observations, and be corroborated. (I am well aware that corroboration requires the refutation of alternatives. But I think it is important—for reasons I discuss later—to note that sometimes hypotheses predict successfully.)

I conclude that predictability and testability both explain the situation better and correct at least one of the errors found in previous discussions. But this conclusion also brings me face-to-face with the criticism that predictability and testability refer only to hypotheses[5-6] and that the familiar criteria (e.g., Hill's) refer only to data.[5]

I must confess that I cannot imagine how it is possible to refer to the testability of a hypothesis without also referring to the relation between its deduced predictions and some carefully chosen observations.[7] Testability obviously "refers" to both. It is also easy to demonstrate that Hill's criteria do not refer exclusively to data. Maclure[5] provides one such counterexample when he discusses "the plausibility of innumerable refuted theories." Another counterexample is the criterion *magnitude of an association*. It explicitly refers both to an observable numerical value and to the hypothetical notion of an association—admittedly a vague notion to many.

However curious my conclusion may seem,[8] the criteria of predictability and testability do explain and correct things better. Therefore, they represent progress in methodologic knowledge. Nevertheless, I will concede that any such progress is precarious.[9] As I show in the next section of this paper, it is more caveat than curiosity that the solution to one problem often leads to a more difficult one, like bouncing off a wall just to crash into another.

Self-Criticism #2: Aren't Things More Complicated With These New Criteria?

The second self-criticism concerns whether the criteria of predictability and testability make our lives more complex. In my opinion, the answer is both *no* and *yes*, for reasons that are best illustrated by analogy.[10]

When you tell someone that you are looking for something unusual or uncommon, a likely reply is "That's like looking for a needle in a haystack." The statement implies that your search may be futile. But keep in mind that things could be much worse. After all, you know what a needle is (and therefore what you're looking for) and you know where the haystack is (and therefore where to look) and finally, you know the needle is there (and therefore that it is worthwhile to search for it).

Our search for explanations in epidemiology straddles both sides of this inferential fence. On the one hand, the careful proposal of a hypothesis and the precise deduction of its observable consequences tells us both what we're looking for and where to look. Things couldn't be simpler. On the other hand, the problem of theoretic diversity—described above—and its solution— the criteria of predictability and testability—also make our lives considerably more complex. There are always a large number of explanatory hypotheses that can be considered in any study, and the greater the number of these possibilities, the greater the number of alternatives that we must try to refute.

To make matters worse, refuting one of these hypotheses— even one with highly testable predictions—is not really like finding that the needle is not in a small portion of the haystack. The search for better explanations of disease is more like a sieve through which the entire haystack must be passed, each sieve providing the mesh to build even finer ones.

Self Criticism #3: Don't I Believe in Criteria If I Advocate Their Use?

I ask this question of myself for two reasons: first, because Greenland reminds us of the importance of beliefs as an initiator of action,[11] and second, because at least one of the contributors to this volume advocates a Popperian approach for epidemiology and yet rejects the use of all inferential criteria.[12]

Belief is a knotty issue for Popperians, because it has strong ties both to inductivism[13] and to an uncritical attitude.[3] One way to look at it is as follows. If I use something in practice—inferential criteria, for example—then I might be willing to say that I "believe" in them. But I think it more precise to say that I have better reasons for tentatively accepting them than for rejecting them. Along with this tentative acceptance comes their trial use in practice followed by an evaluation of their performance.

Evaluation may reveal that these criteria not only work reasonably well, but also that they can withstand criticisms directed at them. Under these circumstances, it is unreasonable to reject them simply on the grounds that they are considered "criteria." No criteria are "true" or "certain." Like all other forms of rational knowledge, inferential criteria are conjectural, uncertain, tentative, and prone to error.

Those who advocate a Popperian approach for epidemiology and yet reject all criteria[12] must be very careful. As I see it, the brightest banner on the bandwagon of Popperianism is refutation. Furthermore, refutation is itself considered a criterion; recently it has been described as necessary but not sufficient for epidemiologic inference.[11,14]

To sum up, I "believe" in the criteria of predictability and testability; I have better reasons for tentatively accepting them than for rejecting them.

Greenland's Criticism

Finally, I think it is wise to focus attention on the important criticism offered by Greenland.[11] With it in hand, I better appreciate the fact that the Popperian epidemiologists have yet to suggest an alternative numerical method. Perhaps one of Petitti's hypothetical graduate students[15] can use this error of omission as a thesis project.

Another important point Greenland makes is that some of the confusion in the philosophical basis of epidemiologic inference stems from our failure to distinguish carefully between the goals, methods, and ethical principles of public health and the goals, methods and ethics of epidemiologic science.

Sometimes we play by different rules, and I agree that the rules of medical technology (within which lies public health) and the rules of medical science, however similar, are not identical. The rules of technology emphasize corroboration; the rules of science emphasize refutation.

Popperians place such great emphasis upon refutation[5] that the importance of corroboration may be easily overlooked. I do not think it heretical of a Popperian perspective to place some importance upon "confirmations" within a bed of refutations of alternatives. Such corroborations are not to be ignored at any rate. We may use them to help us decide the best course of action. May the torch of criticism light the way.

References

1. Williams EN. What *is* the best way for black progress? Washington Post 1985 Dec 1.

2. Skrabanek P. In defense of destructive criticism. Perspectives in Med Biol 1986;30:19–26.

3. Weed DL. Causal criteria and Popperian refutation. In this volume.

4. Susser, M. Falsification, verification and causal inference in epidemiology: reconsiderations in the light of Sir Karl Popper's philosophy. In this volume.

5. Maclure M. Refutation in epidemiology: why else not? In this volume.

6. McIntyre N. The truth, the whole truth and nothing but the truth? In this volume.

7. Weed DL, Selmon M, and Sinks T. Links between categories of interaction. Am J Epidemiol (in press), 1988.

8. Labarthe DR, and Stallones RA. Epidemiologic inference. In this volume.

9. King ML, Jr. *Strength to Love*. New York: Harper and Row 1963:64.

10. Settle T. Induction and probability unfused. In: Schilpp PA, ed. *The Philosophy of Karl Popper*. Library of Living Philosophers, Vol. XIV, Book II. La Salle, Illinois: Open Court 1974:697–749.

11. Greenland S. Probability versus Popper: an elaboration of the insufficiency of current Popperian approaches for epidemiologic analysis. In this volume.

12. Poole C. Induction does not exist in epidemiology, either. In this volume.

13. Weed DL. On the logic of casual inference. Am J Epidemiol 1986;123:965–979.

14. Maclure M. Popperian refutation in epidemiology. Am J Epidemiol 1985;121:345–350.

15. Petitti DB. The implications of alternative views about causal inference for the work of the practicing epidemiologist. In this volume.